What if there's mor

What if it is more c

ABG Interpretation is a challenging skill to learn. Ask several people how to interpret an ABG and you are likely to end up with several approaches. Oakes' ABG Pocket Guide (and the accompanying Instructional Guide) works you through the process of complete interpretation in the context of the patient's clinical presentation.

Putting it together was no easy task, using hundreds of hours of research and study to ensure the best methods were adopted, offering a clear, concise, accurate, and right-to-the-point systematic approach to learning and understanding this essential and often critical diagnostic tool.

By the end of the Instructional Guide you will be proficient at interpreting complex ABGs (including triple disorders!), calculating gaps, and thoughtfully considering causes and potential treatments.

With a focus on just the essentials, this easy to carry, budget friendly, pocket size reference will serve as a vital learning tool, and continuing resource, to Respiratory Care Practitioners, Nurses, Medical Students, Residents, Fellows, PA's, and any other healthcare personnel involved with the interpretation of ABGs.

Let's get started!

Dana Oakes, BA, RRT-NPS

ASSISTANT EDITORS / REVIEWERS

Table of Contents

(continued on next page)

ABG INTERPRETATION =

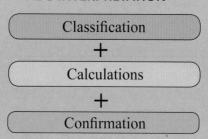

Classification

+

Calculations

+

Confirmation

A. Classification

Respiratory		Metabolic	
Acidosis	Alkalosis	Acidosis	Alkalosis

B. Calculations

Calculate Compensation and Gaps:
Determines whether or not the body is compensating and whether or not other primary disorders exist.

Determine Oxygenation Status

C. Confirmation

Consistency with patient assessment, patient's baseline and check for accuracy: Determines validity of Classification and Calculations

KEYS to INTERPRETATION

1. Initial Technical Classification DOES NOT always equal a definitive ABG interpretation
2. Calculations are always ESSENTIAL
3. Patient assessment is ESSENTIAL
4. Patient BASELINE VALUES are often invaluable
5. Always check for POSSIBLE INACCURACIES in the gas result
6. SERIAL ABGs are often more important than a single ABG
7. ABG interpretation often leads to LIFE and DEATH decisions. Obviously errors are unacceptable!

STEPS OF ABG INTERPRETATION
(See following pages for specific details)

A) Classification

Primary Problem
Step 1. Check pH – Acidosis or Alkalosis?

Primary Cause
Step 2. Check $PaCO_2$ – is Respiratory the primary cause?

Step 3. Check HCO_3^- – is Metabolic the primary cause?

Compensation
Step 4. Is the body compensating?

Initial Classification
Step 5. Technical Classification and/or Functional Classification

B) Calculations
Step 6. Determine if Compensation is Appropriate or are there other Primary Disorders

Step 7. Determine Anion Gap and Bicarbonate Gap

Step 8. Determine Oxygenation

C) Confirmation
Step 9. Systematically Assess Patient

Step 10. Check for Accuracy (errors)

Step 11. **Final Interpretations**

Normal Parameters	Arterial		Mixed Venous	
	Norm	Range	Norm	Range
pH (pHa, pHv̄), units	7.40	7.35-7.45	7.36	7.31-7.41
PCO2 (PaCO2, PV̄CO2), mmHg	40	35-45	46	41-51
PO2 (PaO2, PV̄O2), mmHg*	100	80-100	40	35-42
O2 Sat (SaO2, SV̄O2), %	97%	95-100%	75%	68-77%
HCO3 , mEq/L	24	22-26	24	22-26
TCO2	25	23-27	25	23-27
BE, mEq/L	0	+/- 2	0	+/- 2
O2 content (CaO2, CV̄O2), mL/dL	20	15-24	15	12-15

*21% O2 at sea level

Step 1: Check pH

is pH Normal, Acidosis, or Alkalosis?

Baseline Values (*Start with the patient's baseline when possible*):

pH 7.40, PaCO$_2$ 40 mmHg, HCO$_3$ 24 mEq/L, PaO$_2$ 80 – 100 mmHg

Notes:

For ease of interpretation and consistency, blood gases should be reported in the following sequence: pH/PaCO$_2$/HCO$_3$/O$_2$. (This sequence keeps the first three together – which is the crux of ABG interpretation). Clinically you may find them presented: pH/PaCO$_2$/O$_2$/HCO$_3$

Unless otherwise stated, all values represent spontaneously breathing patients at sea level, with normal body temperature, and breathing room air.

Also, for simplicity, in the remainder of the text the units of measurement will be left off and assumed to be mmHg (torr) for PaO$_2$ and PaCO$_2$ and mEq/L for HCO$_3$ (unless otherwise noted).

In Steps 1, 2, & 3 – one "Key" to accurate ABG interpretation is knowing the patient's baseline values. First, determine from the patient's history if the patient's "normal" baseline values vary from the physiological normals of pH 7.40, PaCO$_2$ 40, and HCO$_3$ 24.

If they do vary, then all ABG interpretation must use the patient's "normal values" (i.e., chronic abnormal baselines, which are maximally compensated), instead of 7.40, 40, and 24.

Example: if a patient with COPD has a baseline pH of 7.34, PaCO$_2$ of 60, and HCO$_3$ of 32, then you should substitute these values for the normal values of 7.40, 40, & 24.

Abnormal Baselines Examples

A. Disease Conditions:

Chronic Respiratory Acidosis: COPD (see page 63), cystic fibrosis (late stage), neuromuscular, sleep disorders, obesity hypoventilation

Chronic Respiratory Alkalosis: Cystic fibrosis (early), pregnancy (3rd trimester), restrictive lung disease (early), some head injuries

Chronic Metabolic Acidosis: Chron. renal failure., renal tub. acidosis

Chronic Metabolic Alkalosis: Chronic systemic steroid/diuretic therapy

B. Newborns:

Normal newborns within the first few hours have gases: pH 7.20 –
7.35, PaCO$_2$ 35 – 55 mmHg, HCO$_3$ 20 – 24, and PaO$_2$ 50-80 mmHg [1].
Following that, newborns, infants, and children have blood gases
that are the same as adults.

[1] *Neonatal/Pediatric Respiratory Care* by Dana Oakes.

C. Venous Blood Gases (VBGs) (specifically pH, PaCO$_2$, and HCO$_3$)

Normal baseline values are pH 7.36 (7.31-7.41), PaCO$_2$ 46 (41-51),
HCO$_3$ same as ABG.

VBGs may often accurately substitute for ABGs. (Mixed venous is
best, peripheral venous may be acceptable if good perfusion in
the region). The value is less cost, risk, and pain to the patient.
VBGs may also be even more indicative of the true cellular envi-
ronment during cardiac arrest than ABGs [2].

Pulse oximetry may substitute for the PaO$_2$ value, when appropriate.

[2] *All You Really Need to Know to Interpret Arterial Blood Gases*, 1999,
L. Martin, Lippincott Williams & Wilkins, p 212.

Step 2: Check PaCO$_2$

is RESPIRATORY the primary cause?

Is PaCO$_2$ normal, ↑, or ↓ ?

Normal PaCO$_2$ = 35-45 mmHg

Respiratory cause = ↑CO$_2$ (hypoventilation) and ↓ pH or
↓CO$_2$ (hyperventilation) and ↑ pH

Note:

If PaCO$_2$ changes from normal in the *opposite direction of pH*, then it is a
Respiratory cause – therefore: a primary (1°) cause.

Think: CO$_2$ = acid   (↑CO$_2$ = ↑ acid = ↓ pH; ↓CO$_2$ = ↓ acid = ↑ pH)
This is due to the hydrolysis reaction:
$$CO_2 + H_2O \leftrightarrow H_2CO_3 \leftrightarrow H^+ + HCO_3$$

Step 3: Check HCO_3

is METABOLIC the primary cause?

Normal HCO_3 = 22-26 mEq/L

Is HCO_3 normal, ↑, or ↓?

Metabolic cause = ↑ HCO_3 and ↑ pH   or   ↓HCO_3 and ↓ pH

Note:
If HCO_3 changes from normal in the *same direction as pH*, then it is a
   Metabolic cause and therefore a primary (1°) cause.
   Think: HCO_3 = base
         (↑HCO_3 = ↑ base = ↑ pH; ↓HCO_3 = ↓ base = ↓ pH)

Step 4: Is the Body Compensating?

If both $PaCO_2$ and HCO_3 are abnormal in the **same direction** then, YES, the body is compensating.

Compensation: $\uparrow PaCO_2$ and $\uparrow HCO_3$
or
$\downarrow PaCO_2$ and $\downarrow HCO_3$

Exception: Hydrolysis (see Step 6)

STEP 5: TECHNICAL CLASSIFICATION

Primary Problem	Primary Cause				Compensation	Initial Classification
Step 1: Check pH	Step 2: Check PaCO2 (35-45)	Is Respiratory 1°?	Step 3: Check HCO3 (22-26)	Is Metabolic 1°?	Step 4: Is the body compensating? (Yes/No)	Step 5: Technical Classification (1)
Alkalosis > 7.45*	↑		↑	Yes	Yes (↑ PaCO2)	PC Metabolic Alkalosis
	N		↑	Yes	-	Metabolic Alkalosis (UC)
	↓	Yes	↑	Yes	-	Mixed Respiratory Alkalosis & Metabolic Alkalosis
	↓	Yes	N,↓		(3)	Respiratory Alkalosis (UC)
	↓	Yes	↓		Yes (↓ HCO3)	PC Respiratory Alkalosis
Normal 7.35-7.45	↑	Yes or compensat.?	↑	Yes or compensat?	Yes (↑ PaCO2)	FC Metabolic Alkalosis (7.41 - 7.45)
	N	Yes or compensat.?	N	Yes or compensat?	Yes (↑ HCO3)	FC Respiratory Acidosis (7.35-7.39)
	N		N		-	Normal or Mixed Disorder (2)
	↓	Yes or compensating?	↓	Yes or compensating?	Yes (↓ PaCO2)	FC Metabolic Acidosis (7.35-7.39)
	↓	Yes or compensating?	↓	Yes or compensating?	Yes (↓ HCO3)	FC Respiratory Alkalosis (7.41-7.45)

						Classification
↑	Yes	←		Yes (↑ HCO₃)		PC Respiratory Acidosis
↑	Yes	N,↑		(3)		Respiratory Acidosis (UC)
↑	Yes	↓	Yes	–		Mixed Respiratory & Metabolic Acidosis
N		↓	Yes	–		Metabolic Acidosis (UC)
↑		↓	Yes	Yes (↓ PaCO₂)		PC Metabolic Acidosis

Acidosis < 7.35 **

NOTES

(1) Technical classification terminology:

UC = Uncompensated (no compensation has occurred). Common usage leaves this designation off.

PC = Partially Compensated (pH has returned part way back to normal range)

FC = Fully Compensated (pH has returned back to normal range)

(2) Mixed Disorder (opposite disorders) = Respiratory acidosis & metabolic alkalosis or respiratory alkalosis & metabolic acidosis (PaCO₂ and HCO₃ go in same direction and "apparent compensation" is greater than expected) (See page 18 for further explanation)

(3) The immediate change in HCO₃ from normal is due to the hydrolysis effect, rather than compensation. (See following pages)

* As pH moves towards 7.8 = ↑ CNS stimulation: irritability, arrhythmias, tetany, convulsions, respiratory arrest, death. Definitive therapy is indicated at pH > 7.6.

** As pH moves towards 7.0 = ↓ CNS stimulation: drowsiness, lethargy, coma, death. Definitive therapy is often considered at pH < 7.15.

Technical Classification	Functional Classification	Compensation Status
UC Respiratory Acidosis	Acute Respiratory Acidosis	**Kidneys:** Either not enough time to begin compensation or the kidneys are compromised
PC Respiratory Acidosis	Chronic Respiratory Acidosis	**Kidneys:** Either not enough time to fully compensate or compensation is maximal (chronic), but pH not back to normal range
FC Respiratory Acidosis	Chronic Respiratory Acidosis	**Kidneys:** Compensation is maximal (chronic) and full – pH is back to normal range (occurs only in very mild disorders)
UC Respiratory Alkalosis	Acute Respiratory Alkalosis	**Kidneys:** Either not enough time to begin compensation or kidneys are compromised
PC Respiratory Alkalosis	Chronic Respiratory Alkalosis	**Kidneys:** Either not enough time to fully compensate or compensation is maximal (chronic), but pH not back to normal range
FC Respiratory Alkalosis	Chronic Respiratory Alkalosis	**Kidneys:** Compensation is maximal (chronic) and full –pH is back to normal range (occurs in most disorders)
UC Metabolic Acidosis	Metabolic Acidosis*	**Respiratory** system is compromised (rare that there is zero compensation) or such a mild change in HCO_3 that any change in $PaCO_2$ is minimal.
PC Metabolic Acidosis	Metabolic Acidosis	**Respiratory:** Compensation is usually immediate and maximal, but pH is not back to normal range
FC Metabolic Acidosis	Metabolic Acidosis	**Respiratory:** This classification essentially *does not exist* because $PaCO_2$ generally does not return pH back to normal range. If pH is normal, there is usually a secondary respiratory disorder at work.
UC Metabolic Alkalosis	Metabolic Alkalosis	**Respiratory :** If there is no compensation, there is usually a secondary respiratory alkalosis
PC Metabolic Alkalosis	Metabolic Alkalosis	**Respiratory:** Compensation is usually immediate and maximal, but pH is not back to normal range
FC Metabolic Alkalosis	Metabolic Alkalosis	**Respiratory:** This class. really *does not exist* because $PaCO_2$ generally does not return pH back to normal range. If pH is normal, there is usually a secondary respiratory disorder at work.

NOTES
Functional Classification = common functional terminology

Functionally, there are only 6 acid-base disorders:
    Respiratory acidosis (acute and chronic)
    Respiratory alkalosis (acute and chronic)
    Metabolic acidosis & Metabolic alkalosis*

* The terms "acute" and "chronic" for metabolic disorders are often omitted because, *functionally*, there is usually no time distinction between acute and chronic metabolic disorders – the respiratory system compensation is usually immediate.
Also, because *all* metabolic disorders are essentially Partially Compensated, all metabolic disorders are simply termed Metabolic Acidosis or Metabolic Alkalosis, without any further descriptive terminology.

Both Technical and Functional Classifications are presented here because, commonly, Respiratory Therapists, Nurses, and various other health care personnel are taught Technical Classifications, and Physicians are commonly taught Functional Classifications. Both methods are correct with each having a particular purpose and function. It is essential that both classification methods be understood for both accuracy of interpretation and accuracy of communication between disciplines.

Example: Technically there could be an uncompensated metabolic acidosis, but functionally it almost never exists.

> A *corrected* blood gas disorder is one in which the pH is returned to normal range by altering the component primarily affected.
> A *compensated* blood gas disorder in one in which the pH is returned towards normal range by altering the component not primarily affected.

Because of the limitations of the lungs or kidneys to "fully" compensate for most alterations of each other (i.e., completely return pH to normal), "*full*" or "*complete*" compensation is more appropriately referred to as *maximal* compensation.

Maximal Compensation = the body has completely compensated all it is designed to compensate – usually pH returns only 50% of the way back towards normal range.

If the disorder is *mild*, maximal compensation may return the pH to within normal range, resulting in a *"full"* compensation (FC).

If the disorder is *moderate to severe*, maximal compensation will only return the pH part way back towards normal range, resulting in a *"partial"* compensation (PC).

Classification Characteristics

Single Disorders	
Respiratory Disorder	pH and $PaCO_2$ go in opposite directions
Metabolic Disorder	pH and HCO_3 go in same direction
Compensating	$PaCO_2$ and HCO_3 go in same direction
Mixed Disorders:*	
Same direction disorders: **Respiratory & Metabolic acidosis** **Respiratory & Metabolic alkalosis**	$PaCO_2$ and HCO_3 go in opposite direction (and change in pH is greater than expected from $PaCO_2$)
Opposite direction disorders: **Respiratory acidosis & Metabolic alkalosis** **Respiratory alkalosis & Metabolic acidosis**	$PaCO_2$ and HCO_3 go in same direction (and compensation is greater than expected)
Mixed Metabolic Disorders	See next pg. & pg. 61

* Triple disorders can also frequently exist (e.g., a Metabolic Acidosis and Metabolic Alkalosis with a Respiratory Acidosis or Respiratory Alkalosis).

Note: Cannot have a quadruple disorder (both Respiratory Acidosis and Respiratory Alkalosis cannot exist at the same time!).

Examples of Mixed Disorders (not all-inclusive)

	Respiratory Acidosis	Respiratory Alkalosis
Metabolic Acidosis	Acute pulmonary edema Cardiac arrest COPD exacerbation and lactic acidosis Poisoning (acidics plus respiratory depression, then lactic acidosis) Respiratory failure and renal failure	Renal insufficiency and CHF or pneumonia Salicylate intoxication Sepsis with hypoxemia and tachypnea Severe liver disease and lactic acidosis Over-ventilation of any patient with metabolic acidosis
Metabolic Alkalosis	COPD with vomiting or diuretics	Critically ill Late pregnancy with vomiting Severe liver disease with vomiting Over-ventilation of a chronic COPD

	Metabolic Acidosis
Metabolic Alkalosis	Renal failure, Alcohol Ketoacidosis (AKA) or Diabetic Ketoacidosis (DKA) with vomiting, diuretics, and/or NG suctioning

Step 6: Determine if Compensation is Appropriate

Are there other Primary Causes?

Note: *Calculations are always required to confirm whether the Technical or Functional Classification is also the Final Interpretation.*

Because of the hydrolysis reaction and the compensatory mechanisms of the body, as one system changes from normal, we can calculate the expected changes that should occur by the body in its attempt to maintain homeostasis.

Changes other than the expected changes indicate the presence of other primary problems.

▶ **Distinguishing between Hydrolysis and Compensation**

There are two primary mechanisms resulting in expected changes - hydrolysis and compensation.

Hydrolysis
Whenever $PaCO_2$ is acutely changed, pH and HCO_3 will also acutely change due to the hydrolysis reaction.

$$CO_2 + H_2O \leftrightarrow H_2CO_3 \leftrightarrow H^+ + HCO_3$$

This reaction takes place primarily in the red blood cell where it is catalyzed by the intracellular enzyme *carbonic anhydrase*.

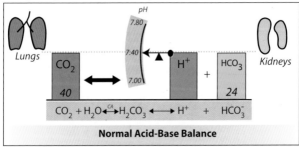

Normal Acid-Base Balance

Acute Respiratory Acidosis

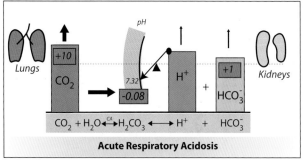

Acute Respiratory Acidosis

Explanation:

For every acute increase of 10 mmHg in $PaCO_2$, pH will decrease 0.08 and HCO_3 will increase 1 mEq.

Acute Respiratory Alkalosis

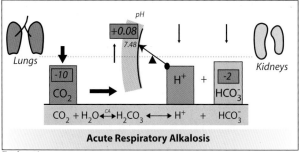

Acute Respiratory Alkalosis

Explanation:

For every acute decrease of 10 mmHg in $PaCO_2$, pH will increase 0.08 and HCO_3 will decrease 2 mEq.

These changes are not considered "compensation", by the kidneys. Technically, it is a buffering, rather than a compensation.

Chronic Respiratory Acidosis

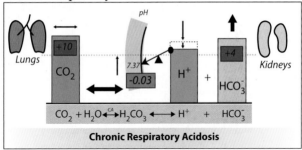

Chronic Respiratory Acidosis

Explanation:

For every chronic increase * of 10 mmHg in $PaCO_2$, the kidneys will respond by increasing the HCO_3 4 mEq/L. This will raise the pH from the acute drop of 0.08 below normal, to only 0.03 below normal.

This is compensation - when one body system responds to counteract the abnormal changes resulting from other body system.

---

* It takes the kidneys, 1- 3 days to maximally compensate for changes in the respiratory CO_2 levels.

Chronic Respiratory Alkalosis

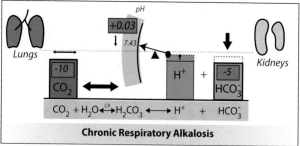

Chronic Respiratory Alkalosis

Explanation:
For every chronic decrease * of 10 mmHg in $PaCO_2$, the kidneys will respond by lowering the HCO_3 5 mEq/L. This will lower the pH from the acute rise of 0.08 above normal, to only 0.03 above normal.

This is compensation - when one body system responds to counteract the abnormal changes resulting from other body system.

---

* It takes the kidneys, 1- 3 days to maximally compensate for changes in the respiratory CO_2 levels.

Metabolic Acidosis

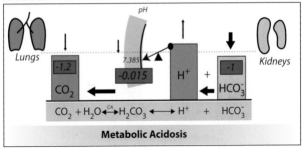

Explanation:
For every decrease of 1 mEq/L of HCO_3, pH will decrease 0.015, and the $PaCO_2$ will decrease 1.2 mmHg.

See next page.

Metabolic Alkalosis

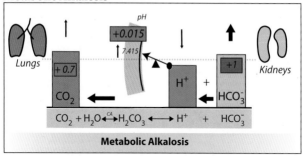

Metabolic Alkalosis

Explanation:

For every increase of 1 mEq/L of HCO_3, pH will increase 0.015, and the $PaCO_2$ will increase 0.7 mmHg. (Note: the $PaCO_2$ change can be highly variable. See section on metabolic alkalosis).

When the kidneys are responsible for an acidosis or alkalosis, the lungs are quick to respond (within minutes) to compensate by either blowing off, or retaining CO_2 (remember: think of CO_2 as an acid) to try and help minimize the metabolic change.

Due to the quickness of the lungs to respond, there is never really any functional distinction between acute vs chronic metabolic alkalosis.

Summary Overview of Hydrolysis and Compensation

	PaCO$_2$	pH	HCO$_3$	Quick Reference Charts:
Respiratory Acidosis				
Acute	↑ 10	↓ 0.08	↑ 1*	See page 31
Chronic	↑ 10	↓ 0.03	↑ 4	
Respiratory Alkalosis				
Acute	↓ 10	↑ 0.08	↓ 2*	See page 44
Chronic	↓ 10	↑ 0.03	↓ 5	

	HCO$_3$	pH †	PaCO$_2$ ‡	Quick Reference:
Metabolic Acidosis	↓ 1	↓ 0.015	↓ 1.2	See page 50
Metabolic Alkalosis	↑ 1	↑ 0.015	↑ 0.7	See page 58

* These changes in HCO$_3$ are due to hydrolysis and not compensation (see below).
† For ease of calculation, for every 1 mEq/L Δ in HCO$_3$, the last digit of pH Δ 1.5
‡ Max PaCO$_2$ = last two digits of pH

Note: All of these changed values are approximations, and the lungs'
changes in response to metabolic conditions are the most variable.
See each corresponding disorder for further details.

There are 2 General Possibilities:

1. **When Compensation is Appropriate (the expected change is seen)**
   This is indicative that *one* and *only one* primary ABG disorder is at
   work and that compensation is normal.

2. **When Compensation is not Appropriate ***

   A. Apparent Over-Compensation (more than expected)

   The body doesn't overcompensate. An apparent overcompensation is
   actually indicative that *another* primary ABG disorder is at work and is
   an "opposite direction" disorder.

   Example: A respiratory acidosis and a metabolic alkalosis. The alkalosis appears to "overcompensate" for the acidosis, but since the body does not overcompensate, it is actually
   not a compensation, but rather another primary disorder.

Note:

This also includes "full" compensation (back to normal range pH) in severe disorders where compensation does not normally return pH to normal – indicative of another primary ABG (opposite direction) disorder (e.g., respiratory alkalosis & metabolic acidosis).

Additionally, an "instant compensation" by the kidneys (which does not occur) is actually an indication of a mixed and opposite disturbance.

B. Absent or Under Compensation (Less then Expected)

This is indicative of three possibilities:

1. The body is unable to compensate due to lung or kidney compromise.

Example: A COPD patient with diabetes mellitus is unable to hyperventilate (compensate) for a metabolic acidosis caused by ketoacidosis (lack of insulin). The inability to hyperventilate could be caused by muscle fatigue or mucous plugging.

2. Insufficient time to compensate.

Example: Respiratory is usually immediate (3-30 min; longer for maximal).The kidneys take 12-24 hours for beginning compensation and up to 2-3 days for full compensation.

3. Another primary ABG disorder is at work and is a "same direction" disorder.

Example: Respiratory acidosis & metabolic acidosis or respiratory alkalosis & metabolic alkalosis

---

> *** NOTE: Allow for normal variations:**
> ± 0.03 pH;
> ± 5 mmHg $PaCO_2$;
> ± 2 mEq/L HCO_3

Step 7: Calculate Anion Gap and Bicarbonate Gap

$$AG = Na^+ - (Cl^- + HCO_3)$$ *see page 52 for explanation*

$$BG = Patient's\ HCO_3 + \Delta AG$$ *see page 62 for explanation*

Step 8: Determine Oxygenation Status

See page 68 for a detailed explanation

Step 9: Systematic Patient Assessment

Check for consistency with patient's condition and baseline.

Note: Patient history and baseline should be pre-assessed even before Step 1. Step 9 is merely a confirmation process.

As with any lab test, we should always treat the patient, not the numbers. Test results can be misleading. Serial ABGs are often more important than a single gas.

A Partial List of Things to Assess:

Patient	Labs	Disease/Disorder	Therapies
History Physical assess. Vital signs Signs & symptoms Chest X-ray (series) CT Scan ECG PFT	Prior ABGs - baseline Blood tests: Hematology Electrolytes Blood glucose BUN Creatinine Lactate	Pathophysiology Exacerbations Drug intake	Drugs Ventilator CPAP/BiPAP High-Flow Oxygen Dialysis (HD, CRRT)

Step 10: Check for Accuracy / Errors

Always check for POSSIBLE INACCURACIES in the blood gas result
See page 94 for details.

Step 11: Final Interpretation

Final Interpretation is often quite different from the initial Technical or
Functional Classification.

> A Quick Reference Guide that recaps these 11 steps can be
> found on the back cover of this book.

Respiratory Acidosis

Definition	PaCO$_2$ > 45 mmHg (Hypercarbia or Hypercapnia)
Cause	Hypoventilation -or- Ventilatory Failure
Compensation	Slow ↑ in HCO$_3$ (Renal ↑ in Base)

Overview of Parameter Changes

	pH	PaCO$_2$	HCO$_3$	K$^+$	Cl$^-$
Uncompensated (acute)	↓	↑	↑*	N	N
Partially Compensated (PC) (chronic)	↓	↑	↑	N	N
Full Compensated (FC) (chronic)**	N	↑	↑↑	N ↑	↓

* The acute change from normal is due to the hydrolysis effect, rather than compensation.
** Rare. Maximal renal compensation commonly results in only partial correction of pH. pH only returns < ½ way back towards normal – unless a very mild respiratory acidosis (See Quick Reference Chart next page).

Determining Compensation

Expected Change in pH and HCO$_3$ for Every 10 mmHg ↑ in PaCO$_2$

	Expected ↓ in pH	Expected ↑ in HCO$_3$
Acute	0.08 *	1
Partially Compensated	0.03-0.08	1-4
Maximally Compensated	0.03	4

*Other references may cite anywhere between 0.05 and 0.1

Equations for Calculations

	Expected pH	Expected HCO₃
Acute	$7.40 - \dfrac{(0.08 \times \Delta PaCO_2)}{10}$	$24 + \dfrac{(1 \times \Delta PaCO_2)}{10}$
Chronic (maximally compensated)	$7.40 - \dfrac{(0.03 \times \Delta PaCO_2)}{10}$	$24 + \dfrac{(4 \times \Delta PaCO_2)}{10}$

Note: Partial compensation is not normally calculated, but rather determined to be somewhere between the calculated acute and maximally compensated values.

Example: Acute Respiratory Acidosis with a PaCO₂ of 60 mmHg

Expected pH	Expected HCO₃
$7.40 - \dfrac{(0.08 \times \underline{60-40})}{10}$	$24 + \dfrac{(1 \times \underline{60-40})}{10}$
$7.40 - 0.16 = 7.24$	$24 + 2 = 26$

Quick Reference Chart - Expected Values

PaCO₂	Acute		Partially Compensated	Fully (or Maximally) Compensated	
	pH*	HCO₃	pH/HCO₃	pH	HCO₃
90	7.00	29		7.25	44
85	7.04				
80	7.08	28		7.28	40
75	7.12				
70	7.16	27	← between →	7.31	36
65	7.20				
60**	7.24	26		7.34**	32
55	7.28				
50	7.32	25		7.37	28
45	7.36				
40	7.40	24		7.40	24

* From a normal pH of 7.40. Allow ± 0.03 for normal patient and machine variation.
** Note: Above a PaCO₂ of 60 mmHg, pH does not return to within normal range, even with maximal renal compensation.

Signs & Symptoms of Acute Respiratory Acidosis

(relative order of appearance, and varies with severity)

Hypoxemia *(due to alveolar air equation)*	Vasodilation (diaphoresis, flushing)	Somnolence
		Tremors
Tachypnea	Headache	Slurred speech
Dyspnea	Confusion	Hallucination
Anxiety, agitation	Disorientation	Psychosis
Tachycardia	Bradypnea	Stupor
Hypertension (early)	Hypotension (late)	Convulsions
Bounding pulses	Drowsiness	Coma
Diaphoresis	Lethargy	Death

Signs & Symptoms of Chronic Respiratory Acidosis

Morning headache, Mild irritability, Lethargy, Disturbed sleep patterns

	Physiological Effects	Clinical Manifestations
Cardiopulm. System	↓ myocardial contractility ↑or↓ myocardial irritability Pulmonary vascular constriction Systemic vasodilation	Arrhythmias Heart failure, ↓ CO Flushed skin color /diaphoresis Pulmonary hypertension Systemic hypotension
Central Nervous System (CNS)	Depressed cortical function ↑ cerebral perfusion*, dilated cerebral vessels, ↑ intracranial pressure (ICP) ↑or ↓ resp. center activity	Disoriented, confusion, somnolence, coma Focal neuro signs, NM irritab. Headache, ↑ CSF Press, ↑ ICP Hyperventilation (if metabolic) Hypoventilation (if respiratory)
Renal & Metabolic	↑ serum Cl^- and K^+ (early) ↑ excretion of Cl^- and K^+ (later) Reabsorption of HCO_3	Hyper/hypochloremia Hyperkalemia ↑ urine K^+ Nausea, vomiting

* Cerebral blood flow (CBF) may double with acute ↑ $PaCO_2$. A slow increase (permissive hypercapnia) is tolerated well.

Note: In chronic Respiratory Acidosis (e.g., COPD), CBF has normalized, so ↓ $PaCO_2$ to "normal" (40 mmHg) may significantly ↓ CBF (See respiratory alkalosis).

Causes of Respiratory Acidosis
(Alveolar Hypoventilation, Ventilatory Failure)

Pulmonary	Chest Wall	CNS Depression	Metabolic (excessive CO_2 production)*
Acute airway obstruction: Aspiration Bronchiolitis Bronchoconstriction Croup Cystic Fibrosis Edema/inflammation Epiglottitis Foreign objects Laryngospasm Post-extubation Secretions, etc. Smoke/chemicals *Asthma, COPD:* Acute exacerbation Late stages *Decreased functioning of lung tissue (severe):* ARDS, Atelectasis, Fibrosis, Pneumonia, Pulmonary edema, Pulmonary embolism *Sleep apnea* (obstructive)	*Restrictive disorders (severe):* Flail chest Kyphoscoliosis Obesity hypoventilation Rib fracture Severe burns Trauma **Intrathoracic** Empyema Hemothorax Pleural disease/ effusion Pneumothorax	Cerebral ischemia CVA (infarcts) *Drugs:* alcohol intoxication, anesthetics, barbiturates, benzodiazepines, cocaine/ heroin, methadone, mor-phine/sedatives, narcotics, propofol, propoxyphene, tranquilizers Increased ICP (hypoxic brain) Infection Lesions/tumors Metabolic alkalosis (CSF) O_2 therapy (in COPD) Pickwickian syndrome Primary hypoventilation (Ondine's curse) Sleep apnea (central) Stroke Trauma (head)	Burns (severe) Fever High carbohydrate diet $NaHCO_3$ admin Sepsis Total parenteral nutrition (TPN) *(Con't Next Page)*

Neuromuscular	Cardiovascular	Other
ALS	Cardiac arrest ($\downarrow$ CO)	Air trapping
Drugs: antibiotics, anticholinesterase, curare/non-depolarizers, dexamethonium, nerve gases, succinylcholine	CHF with pulmonary edema	Fatigue
	Congenital heart disease	Excess O_2 in chronic CO_2 retainers
	Hypovolemia	Hypothyroidism
Electrolyte imbalance	Shock	Malnutrition
Guillian-Barré syndrome	Thromboemboli	Mechanical hypoventilation
High spinal injury/disease		Post-op complications
Multiple sclerosis		
Muscular dystrophy		
Myasthenia gravis		
Myotonia		
Phrenic nerve injury		
Poisons/toxins: botulism, mushrooms, paraquat, petroleum distillates		
Poliomyelitis, Polymyositis		
Potassium and phosphate depletion		
Rabies, SLE		
Status epilepticus		
Tetanus		

* Only a factor when the patient's ability to blow off the excess CO_2 becomes compromised (prolonged time or pulmonary dysfunction).

Management of Respiratory Acidosis

Problem – Hypoventilation (↑ $PaCO_2$ → ↓ pH)
Goal – Improve ventilation and normalization of pH by ↓ $PaCO_2$ *

* Treat the primary ABG disorder. Secondary changes (i.e., compensations) will usually correct themselves after the primary disorder is corrected (unless the body is unable to).

Normalization should always aim for the patient's normal baseline values. Do not over correct (especially in patients with abnormal baselines).

Therapy

Correct	Compensate
Correct underlying problem of hypoventilation (acute or chronic *)	N/A

* Contrary to conditions of Acute Respiratory Acidosis, the underlying causes of Chronic Respiratory Acidosis can only rarely be resolved (e.g., COPD; see "ABGs in COPD" page 63).

Therapies Used to Correct Pulmonary Problems*

Aerosol and Humidity Therapy Airway Management Bronchial Hygiene Therapy Bronchodilator Therapy Lung Expansion Therapy	Oxygen Therapy (see page 68) Systemic steroids Noninvasive Positive Pressure Ventilation (NPPV) ** Mech. Ventilation (See next page) **

* See Oakes' ***Clinical Practitioner's Pocket Guide To Respiratory Care*** for details of management therapies.

** See Oakes' ***Ventilator Management Pocket Guide*** for detailed management.

For detailed management of neonates and children, see Oakes'
  Neonatal/Pediatric Respiratory Care: A Critical Care Pocket Guide.

Ventilator Management of Respiratory Acidosis

Indications for Ventilatory Support

Indications	Description	Examples
Acute Respiratory Failure (ARF)	Inability of a patient to maintain adequate PaO_2, $PaCO_2$, and potentially pH.	Hypoxemic Resp. Failure Hypercapnic Resp. Failure (see next page)
Impending Respiratory Failure	Respiratory failure is imminent in spite of therapies. Commonly defined as: Patient is barely maintaining (or experiencing gradual deterioration) of normal blood gases at the expense of significant WOB (see figure next page)	N-M disease Status asthmaticus
Prophylactic Ventilatory Support	Clinical conditions in which there is a high risk of future respiratory failure. Ventilatory support is instituted to ↓ WOB, minimize O_2 consumption and hypoxemia, reduce cardiopulmonary stress, and/or control airway with sedation.	Brain injury Heart muscle injury Major surgery Shock (prolonged) Smoke injury
Hyper-ventilation Therapy	Ventilatory support is instituted to control and manipulate $PaCO_2$ to lower than normal levels.	Acute head injury

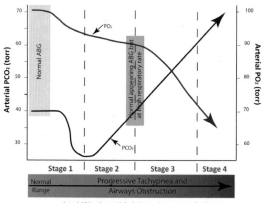

Arterial blood gas, ABG, during various stages of asthma.

Two Types of Acute Respiratory Failure

	Hypoxemic Resp. Failure	Hypercapnic Resp. Failure
Names	Type I ARF, Lung Failure Oxygenation Failure Respiratory Insufficiency	Type II ARF, Pump Failure Ventilatory Failure
Def.	The failure of lungs and heart to provide adequate O_2 to meet metabolic needs.	The failure of the lungs to eliminate CO_2
Criteria	$PaO_2 < 60$ mm Hg on $FIO_2 \geq .50$ or $PaO_2 < 40$ mm Hg on any FIO_2 $SaO_2 < 90$	Acute ↑ in $PaCO_2 > 50$ mm Hg or Acutely above normal baseline in COPD with concurrent ↓ in pH < 7.30
Basic Causes	R-L shunt V/Q mismatch Alveolar hypoventilation Diffusion defect Inadequate FIO_2	Pump failure (drive, muscles, WOB) ↑ CO_2 production R-L shunt ↑ deadspace

Respiratory Acidosis 37

Indications for Ventilatory Assistance Based on ABG Parameters

Parameter*	Normal Value	Ventilator Assistance Indicated
Ventilation		
$PaCO_2$	35-45 mmHg	50-55 mmHg or acute ↑ from patient's baseline (e.g., COPD)
pH	7.35 - 7.45	< 7.25
Oxygenation		
PaO_2	80 - 100 mmHg (room air)	< 50 mmHg (room air) < 60 mmHg (50% O_2) < 200 mmHg (100% O_2)
SaO_2	> 95%	< 85%
PaO_2/PAO_2	0.8-0.9	< 0.15
PaO_2/FIO_2	> 400	< 300
Qs/QT (shunt)	< 5%	> 20%

* No one parameter or set of parameters has been proven to be an absolute indication for MV. Clinical judgment is to take precedence over objective parameters and trends are far more important than absolute values.

See Oakes's *Ventilator Management Pocket Guide* for other detailed criteria, such as mechanical capabilities.

Improving Ventilation   (Correcting / Adjusting $PaCO_2$ and pH)

Goal: Maintain adequate gas exchange using safe volumes and pressures.

Principle: Adequacy of ventilation is determined by delivered $\dot{V}_E$ and assessed by $PaCO_2$ and pH.

$PaCO_2$ and the resultant pH ≈ total ventilation, deadspace, and CO_2 production and are changed by altering $\dot{V}_E$, $\dot{V}_D$, and/or CO_2 production.

Note: Ventilation management should be aimed at normalizing pH, rather than $PaCO_2$ (except when permissive hypercapnia with low pH is being allowed).

Situation: ↑ $PaCO_2$ with ↓pH   (Acute Respiratory Acidosis)

Problem: ↓$\dot{V}_E$	In Volume Ventil.	In Pressure Ventil.
Solution: ↑$\dot{V}_E$ New $\dot{V}_E$ = current $\dot{V}_E$ x ($PaCO_2$/ desired $PaCO_2$)	↑$\dot{V}_E$ by: 1) ↑ V_T (up to 10-12 mL/kg, providing P_{Plat} < 30 cm H_2O)* 2) ↑ f (if V_T and P_{plat} are already high)	↑$\dot{V}_E$ by: 1) ↑ set pressure (PIP, P_{limit}) 2) ↑ T_I (if short)

* Except in ARDS

Additional Strategies
1) Increase V_{Tspont}:
   A) Pressure support ventilation
   B) Bronchodilation
   C) Increase ET tube size
   D) Respiratory muscle conditioning
   E) Improve nutritional support
   F) Decrease sedation

2) Decrease mechanical V_D:
   A) Use low compliance circuit
   B) Cut ET tube shorter
   C) Tracheostomy
3) High Frequency Ventilation
4) Permissive Hypercapnia

Situation: $\uparrow PaCO_2$ with $\downarrow$ pH (Despite Adequate or High $\dot{V}_E$)

Possible Problems

$\uparrow$ Deadspace (V_D/V_T)	$\uparrow CO_2$ Production
Possible Causes: Air trapping High I:E ratio (e.g., 3:1) Low $\dot{V}_I$ Pulmonary emboli or hypoperfusion Uneven gas distribution (lung pathology)	*Possible Causes:* Burns Fever Hyperthyroidism Multiple surgeries Multiple trauma Sepsis
Possible Solutions: Increase flow Decrease I:E ratio Reposition patient Heliox?	*Possible Solutions:* Correct primary cause Note: Increasing $\dot{V}_E$ further may lead to air trapping and auto-PEEP PSV may be helpful to $\downarrow$WOB

Deadspace Assessment

Minute Ventilation ($\dot{V}_E$) = $\dot{V}_A$ + $\dot{V}_D$

$PaCO_2 \approx 1/\dot{V}_A$ ($\uparrow\dot{V}_A \rightarrow \downarrow PaCO_2$; $\downarrow\dot{V}_A \rightarrow \uparrow PaCO_2$)
$PaCO_2 \approx \dot{V}_D$ ($\uparrow\dot{V}_D \rightarrow \uparrow PaCO_2$; $\downarrow\dot{V}_D \rightarrow \downarrow PaCO_2$)

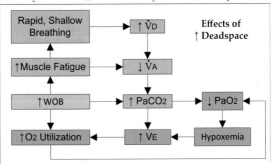

Types of Deadspace

	Types	Description	Causes
Physiological	*Mechanical*	Air outside body that is rebreathed	Added ventilator tubing (between wye and patient) Paper Bag
	Anatomical	Conducting airways	Rapid, shallow breathing increases the proportion of VDanatomical: ↑ WOB, anxiety CNS malfunction
	Alveolar	Alveoli w/o perfusion (Deadspace unit; V/0) Alveoli with ↓ perfusion (Deadspace effect; V/↓Q)	*No perfusion:* Cardiac arrest Pulmonary emboli *↓ Perfusion:* Alveolar overinflation – Airtrapping, MV, PEEP *↑ PVR –* Acidemia, ↓ PAO₂, ↓ PaO₂ Shock *↓ Perfusion surface area:* Emphysema

Deadspace vs. Shunt

	Deadspace	Shunt
↑ $\dot{V}_E$	No significant Δ in $PaCO_2$	↓ $PaCO_2$
↑ FIO_2	↑ PaO_2	No significant Δ in PaO_2
$P(a\text{-}A)CO_2$	↑	No effect
$P(A\text{-}a) O_2$	No effect	↑

See pages 74, and 79 for further information on shunts.

Respiratory Acidosis

Troubleshooting

Checklist for Worsening Respiratory Acidosis or Alkalosis in Mechanically Ventilated Patients

Patient-Related Causes	
Airway problems: Bronchospasm/edema ET tube dislocation (pharynx, esophagus, carina, Right mainstem placement) ET tube kink (bending or biting) ET tube cuff (leak, rupture, herniation) Secretions/obstructions T-E fistula **Lung problems:** Atelectasis Auto-PEEP B-P fistula Pneumothorax **Cardiovascular problems:** CHF Fluid imbalance Innominate artery rupture MI Pulmonary edema Pulmonary embolism	**Altered respiratory drive:** Anxiety Delirium Drugs Excessive carbohydrate load Fear Fever Inadequate nutritional support Pain Stress **Other Causes:** Abdominal distension Altered patient position Drug-induced problems Electrolyte imbalance
	Ventilator-Related Causes
	Inadequate or altered settings: Inadequate FIO_2 ($\downarrow PaO_2$) Inadequate ventilatory support ($\uparrow PaCO_2$, $\uparrow WOB$) Improper sensitivity setting Leak/disconnection Malfunction (ventilator, circuit, humidifier, valves) Patient-ventilator asynchrony

See Oakes's *Ventilator Management: A Bedside Reference Guide* for much more detail in managing patients on mechanical ventilators.

Respiratory Alkalosis

Definition	$PaCO_2 < 35$ mmHg (Hypocarbia or Hypocapnia)
Cause	Hyperventilation
Compensation	Slow $\downarrow$ in HCO_3 (Renal $\downarrow$ in Base)

Overview of Parameter Changes

	pH	$PaCO_2$	HCO_3	K^+	Cl^-
Uncompensated (acute)	$\uparrow$	$\downarrow$	$\downarrow$*	N	N
Partially compensated (PC) (chronic)	$\uparrow$	$\downarrow$	$\downarrow$	N	N
Full Compensated (FC) chronic**	N	$\downarrow$	$\downarrow\downarrow$	N$\downarrow$	$\uparrow$

* The acute change from normal is due to the hydrolysis effect, rather than compensation.

Determining Compensation

Expected Change in pH and HCO_3 for Every 10 mmHg $\downarrow$ in $PaCO_2$

	Expected $\uparrow$ in pH	Expected $\downarrow$ in HCO_3
Acute	0.08 *	2
Partially Compensated	0.03-0.08	2-5
Maximally Compensated	0.03	5

*Some references use 0.1

Equations for Calculations

	Expected pH	Expected HCO$_3$
Acute	$7.40 + (0.08 \times \dfrac{\Delta \, PaCO_2}{10})$	$24 - (2 \times \dfrac{\Delta \, PaCO_2}{10})$
Chronic (maximally compensated)	$7.40 + (0.03 \times \dfrac{\Delta \, PaCO_2}{10})$	$24 - (5 \times \dfrac{\Delta \, PaCO_2}{10})$

Note: Partial compensation is not normally calculated, but rather determined to be somewhere between the calculated acute and maximally compensated values.

Example: Acute Respiratory Alkalosis with a PaCO$_2$ of 20 mmHg

Expected pH	Expected HCO$_3$
$7.40 + (0.08 \times \dfrac{40-20}{10})$	$24 - (2 \times \dfrac{60-40}{10})$
$7.40 + 0.16 = 7.56$	$24 - 4 = 20$

Quick Reference Chart - Expected Values

PaCO$_2$	Acute		Partially Compensated	Fully (or Maximally) Compensated	
	pH*	HCO$_3$	pH/HCO$_3$	pH	HCO$_3$
40	7.40	24		7.40	24
35	7.44	23			
30	7.48	22		7.43	19
25	7.52	21	← between →		
20**	7.56	20		7.46	14
15	7.60	19			
10	7.64	18		7.49	9

* From a normal pH of 7.40. Allow ± 0.03 for normal patient and machine variation.
** Note: Rarely is PaCO$_2$ 20 mmHg or less. Therefore, full renal compensation usually returns pH to within normal range.

Caution: When acute Respiratory Alkalosis appears to be returning to "normal" (i.e., PaCO$_2$ increases back towards 40 mmHg and pH decreases back towards 7.40), *but the patient is not improving or worsening in symptoms* (e.g., severe asthma attack), then the "return to normal" is probably Respiratory Acidosis (hypoventilation) occurring due to fatigue. *This is a danger sign of impending ventilatory failure.* See diagram on page 37.

Signs & Symptoms of Acute Respiratory Alkalosis

(Relative order of appearance and varies with severity)

Early:
Hyperventilation, dyspnea, light headedness, dizziness, paresthesia (numbness or tingling in extremities), chest pain or tightness
Anxiety, nervousness
Tachycardia, palpitations
↑ K$^+$

Late:
Confusion,
↓ concentration
Euphoria
Hyperactive reflexes → tetany
Hallucinations
Seizures
↓ K$^+$
Stupor

	Physiological Effects	Clinical Manifestations
Cardiopulmon. System	↑ myocardial irritability Bronchoconstriction Pulmonary vasodilation Coronary vasoconstriction Systemic vasoconstriction	Arrhythmias Dyspnea ↓ PVR ↑ HR, palpitations Chest pain Pale skin color
Central Nervous System (CNS)	↑ excitability and NM irritability Cerebral vasoconstriction (↓ CBF, ↓ cerebral edema)* ↑or ↓ respiratory center activity	Anxiety, nervousness, light-headedness, tingling / numbness, ↑reflexes, seizures, tetany ↓ CSF pressure, ↓ ICP Hyperventilation
Renal & Metabolic	↓ serum Cl$^-$ and K$^+$ ↓ excretion of K$^+$ Excretion of HCO$_3$	Hyper/hypochloremia Hypokalemia ↓ urine K$^+$

* Cerebral blood flow (CBF) may ↓ 50% with PaCO$_2$ ↓ of 10 mmHg PaCO$_2$.

Causes of Respiratory Alkalosis (Alveolar Hyperventilation) *

CNS Disorders	Metabolic	↓ Diaph. Movement
Brain tumors CVA (infarct) **Drugs**: catecholamines, epinephrine, nicotine, progesterone, respiratory stimulants, salicylate poisoning (early), xanthines Infections (G- sepsis) Lesions (meningitis, encephalitis) Metabolic acidosis (CSF) **Psychogenic**: anxiety, fear, hyperventilation syndromes, neurosis, pain, psychosis Trauma	Hypothermia Bacteremia (sepsis) Exercise Fever Hepatic failure (coma) Hyperthyroidism Metabolic acidosis	Abdominal distension (Ascites) Obesity Pregnancy (late)
	Pulmonary	**Cardiovascular**
	ARDS (early) Asthma (early) Atelectasis (early) COPD (early) Pneumonia (early) Pulmonary burns Pulmonary edema Pulmonary embolism Restrictive disorders	Anemia CHF Myocardial Infarction Pulmonary embolism Shock
		Other
Hypoxemia = MOST COMMON CAUSE		High Altitude Respiratory Therapist (Ventilator settings)*

*We should be acutely aware of ventilator settings that are causing a patient to be alkalotic. **Hint**: You will notice that the patient is not overbreathing the ventilator settings (the set minute ventilation is greater than the patient's needed minute ventilation)

Continued or prolonged severe Respiratory Alkalosis may rapidly progress to Respiratory Acidosis due to muscle fatigue from hyperventilation (especially in pulmonary compromised patients).

Management of Respiratory Alkalosis

Problem – Hyperventilation ($\downarrow PaCO_2 \rightarrow \uparrow$ pH)
Goal – Reduce ventilation and normalization of pH by $\uparrow PaCO_2$ *

* Treat the primary ABG disorder. Secondary changes (i.e., compensations) will usually correct themselves after the primary disorder is corrected (unless the body is unable).

Therapy

Correct	Compensate *
Correct underlying problem (acute or chronic):	*Decrease* HCO_3: Acetazolamide (controversial), hemodialysis with low HCO_3 bath
Correct hypoxemia** Coaching for proper breathing (slow and deep) Pain medication for pain Sedation for hysteria Normalize body temp for hypothermia	*Increase* $PaCO_2$: Re-breathing into a closed system (paper bag) If severe or prolonged - controlled ventilation with mechanical ventilation, with or without sedation/paralysis.

* Usually done only when pH > 7.55
** Although hypoxemia is the most common reason for Respiratory Alkalosis, and O_2 therapy can correct the hypoxemia and resulting hyperventilation, the underlying cause of the hypoxemia must be found and treated.

Chronic Respiratory Alkalosis:

If mild, such as in late pregnancy, the alkalosis poses a low risk to health and produces few or no symptoms and therefore, generally requires no correction.
Some patients may require breathing exercises and training in proper breathing.

Ventilator Management of Respiratory Alkalosis

Correction of Respiratory Alkalosis from Hyperventilation

Situation: $\downarrow PaCO_2$ and $\uparrow pH$ (Uncompensated Respiratory Alkalosis)

Problem	In Volume Ventilation	In Pressure Ventilation
Excessive $\dot{V}A$ BY VENT. Solution: $\downarrow \dot{V}A$ by $\downarrow$ vent $\dot{V}E$	$\downarrow f$: Desired f = known $PaCO_2$ x (known f / desired $PaCO_2$) Desired $\dot{V}E$ = known $PaCO_2$ x (known $\dot{V}E$ / desired $PaCO_2$) $\downarrow V_T$: Desired V_T = known $PaCO_2$ x (known V_T / desired $PaCO_2$)	$\downarrow f$: Desired f = known $PaCO_2$ x (known f / desired $PaCO_2$) $\downarrow$ Set pressure: Desired set pressure = known V_T x (known set pressure / desired V_T)
Excessive $\dot{V}A$ BY PATIENT	If patient is on A/C, decreasing f of mandatory breaths may have no effect. If $\downarrow V_T$ and patient increases f then: 1) Try Pressure Support Ventilation (maybe SIMV?) 2) Sedate (especially in patients with extreme agitation, fear, pain, or $\uparrow$WOB) 3) Add mech. deadspace (unlikely clinically today) **If patient is hyperventilating due to hypoxemia – correct hypoxemia. Do not try to correct hyperventilation without first correcting hypoxemia.**	

Note: Ventilation management should be aimed at normalizing pH, rather than $PaCO_2$.

Troubleshooting

Checklist for Worsening Respiratory Alkalosis in Mechanically Ventilated Patients (See page 42)

Metabolic Acidosis

Definition	$HCO_3 < 22$ mEq/L
Cause	↑ Acid or ↓ Base
Compensation	Hyperventilation

Overview of Parameter Changes

	pH	$PaCO_2$	HCO_3	K^+	Cl^-
Uncompensated*	↓	↓	↓	↑	↑
Partially Compensated (PC) (chronic)	↓	↓	↓	↑	↑
Full Compensated (FC) (chronic)**	N	↓	↓↓	N	N

* Rare. There is usually some degree of immediate (10 – 30 min) respiratory compensation (hyperventilation), unless there is respiratory impairment. Hence, there is usually no distinction between acute and chronic.
    If there is no compensation, then the respiratory system is compromised.
    In rapid changes of HCO_3, respiratory compensation may take 12-24 hours.

** This classification essentially does not exist because $PaCO_2$ generally does not return pH back to normal range (usually only ½ way back). If pH is normal, there is usually a secondary respiratory disorder at work.

Determining Compensation

Expected Change in pH and HCO_3 for Every 1 mEq/L ↓ in HCO_3

	Expected ↓ in pH	Expected ↓ in $PaCO_2$ (mmHg)
Acute and Chronic	0.015	1.2-1.5 (max) **

* For ease of calculation, for every 1 mEq/L ↓ in HCO_3, the last digit of pH ↓ 1.5.
** Maximal compensation: $PaCO_2$ = last two digits of pH

Equations

Expected $PaCO_2 = [1.5 \times HCO_3] + 8 \ (\pm 2)$ (Winter's Formula)
    or
Expected $PaCO_2 = HCO_3 + 15$
    or
Expected $PaCO_2 =$ last two digits of pH (maximal compensation)

Quick Reference Chart - Expected Values

HCO_3	↓ pH*	↓ $PaCO_2$ (max) **
24	7.40	40
22	7.37	38 (37)
20	7.34	35 (34)
18	7.31	33 (31)
16	7.28	30 (28)
14	7.25	28 (25)
12	7.22	26 (22)
10	7.19	23 (19)
8	7.16	21 (16) ***
6	7.13	18 (13)
4	7.10	16 (10)
2	7.07	13 (7)

* From a normal pH of 7.40
** Maximal compensation: $PaCO_2 =$ last two digits of pH.
  Compensation is usually immediate (10-30 min) and maximal unless pulmo
    nary impairment. If there is pulmonary impairment, then $PaCO_2$ levels
    will be proportionally higher than expected.

If $PaCO_2$ levels are higher than expected, there is a secondary respiratory
  acidosis.
If $PaCO_2$ levels are lower than expected, there is a secondary respiratory
  alkalosis.

*** Note: Rarely does hyperventilation occur below a $PaCO_2$ of 15 (6-8 mmHg
in children).

Signs & Symptoms of Metabolic Acidosis

Air hunger:
  Hyperventilation (compensation)
  Dyspnea
  Hyperpnea
  Tachypnea
  Kussmaul's respiration
    (Diabetic ketoacidosis)

Dry skin & mucous
membranes
Weakness & muscle
fatigue
Restlessness
Hypotension
Lethargy

Seizures
Stupor
Coma
Death

	Physiological Effects	Clinical Manifestations
Cardiopulmonary System	Respiratory distress ↓ strength of respiratory muscles ↓ cardiac contractility, arteriolar vasodilation, veno-constriction, and centralization of blood volume	Hyperventilation Dyspnea ↑ muscle fatigue ↓ CO, ↓ BP Arrhythmias Systemic vasodilation
Central Nervous System	Progressive obtundation	Lethargy, Seizures, Stupor Coma, Death
Renal & Metabolic	↑metabolic demands Hyperkalemia	↑ K^+

Two Types of Metabolic Acidosis

1. *Anion Gap Metabolic Acidosis* (↑ acid) : ↑ acid → ↑ AG

2. *Non-Anion Gap Metabolic Acidosis* (↓ base) : ↓ HCO_3^- → ↑ Cl^-
   (Also called Hyperchloremic Metabolic Acidosis)

What is the Anion Gap ?

$AG = Na^+ - (Cl^- + HCO_3^-)$
    = the difference between measured cations (+) and anions (−)
    = unmeasured ions
Normal AG = 12 (± 4) mEq/L

Note: Some clinicians, notably nephrologists, add potassium into the formula; $AG = (Na^+ + K^+) - (Cl^- + HCO_3^-)$, giving a normal value of 16 (12–20) mEq/L.

Normal

Cations
Na⁺ 140

Anions		
AG 12	HCO₃ 24	Cl⁻ 104

1. Anion Gap Metabolic Acidosis = ↑ anion gap (AG) from an ↑ acid

↑ acid = ↑ unmeasured anions = ↑ AG which causes a
        corresponding ↓ HCO₃
A true AG Metabolic Acidosis = ↑ anion gap of > 16 (↓ HCO₃ < 20).
In pure AG Metabolic Acidosis: ↑ AG should = ↓ HCO₃ (a 1:1 ratio)

AG	HCO₃
24	12
22	14
20	16
18	18
16	20
14	22
12	24

If not a 1:1 ratio, then not a pure AG cause;
consider a mixed metabolic disorder (See
page 61)

Example

Normal AG	Increased AG
$AG = Na^+ - (Cl^- + HCO_3)$	$AG = Na^+ - (Cl^- + HCO_3)$
$= 140 - (104 + 24)$	$= 140 - (104 + \downarrow 16)$
$= 140 - 128$	$= 140 - 120$
$= 12\ (\pm 4)$ *	$= \uparrow 20$

* Note: Normal AG = ½ HCO_3

Cations		
Na^+ 140		
Anions		
AG ↑20	HCO_3 ↓16	Cl^- 104

2. **Non- Anion Gap Metabolic Acidosis** = Decreased base (↓ HCO_3) (which causes ↑ Cl^-, anion gap stays the same)

Commonly called ***Hyperchloremic Metabolic Acidosis***

Cations		
Na^+ 140		
Anions		
AG 12	HCO_3 ↓14	Cl^- ↑114

Causes of Anion Gap Metabolic Acidosis (↑ Acid →↑ AG)

↑ Acid Production	↑ Acid Addition	↓ Acid Excretion
Organic acids:	Toxins:	Dehydration
	CO poison, cyanide,	Hypoaldosteronism
↑ Lactic acid *	ethylene glycol	Renal failure
(*most common cause*) (> 5mM/L)	(antifreeze), INH, isoniazid, methanol	(azotemic ketoacidosis)
	(Sterno), nitroprusside,	($\uparrow$ BUN > 40 mg/dL
↑ Ketoacidosis **	paraldehyde, propylene	& ↑ creatinine > 4
(common cause)	glycol, salicylates (late),	mg/dL)
	toluene (paint thinner)	
↑ PO_4		
↑ SO_4		Trauma
↑ Proteins (hyperalbuminemia; > 4.4 g/dl)	Drugs:	
	Penicillin	

* Causes of ↑ Lactic acid (Lactic acidosis)

Type A - Hypoxic Lactic Acidosis		Type B - Non-Hypoxic LA
Hypoxemia (*most common cause*) (any disorder causing anaerobic metabolism)		Diabetes
		Infection(severe)(AIDS)
		Leukemia
		Liver failure
Under delivery of O_2 *to the tissue cells:*	*Over consumption of* O_2 *by the tissue cells:*	Neoplasms
		Pancreatitis
Anemia (severe)		Renal failure
Asthma (severe)	Muscle fatigue	Thiamine deficiency
Carbon monoxide poisoning	Seizures (rhabdomyolysis)	
Cardiac arrest	Sepsis	
Cyanide poisoning	Shivering (severe)	
Hemoglobinopathies	Severe exercise	
Shock		

** Causes of ↑ Keto acids (ketoacidosis)
   AKA: Alcohol ketoacidosis (common: alcohol + starvation)
   DKA: Diabetic ketoacidosis (lack of insulin) (most common cause)
   (glucose > 300 mg% and confirmed by "ketones" in the urine or blood)
   SKA: Starvation ketoacidosis (3-14 days)

Cause of ↓ Anion Gap (↓ acid below normal)

↓ Protein
(hypoalbuminemia; < 4.4 g/dL)

For every 1 g/dL decline in serum albumin <4.4 g/dL, a 2.5 mEq/L reduction in AG occurs.

Causes of Non-anion Gap (Hyperchloremic) Metabolic Acidosis
(↓ Base)

↓ Base (loss of HCO$_3$)	

↑ Kidney Excretion:
Renal tubular acidosis
  (↑ HCO$_3$ excretion)
Urinary diversion or obstruction
CaCl, MgSO4
 	
Intestinal loss:
Diarrhea (*most common cause*)
  (incl. laxative abuse)
Enteric drainage tubes
Ileostomy
Small bowel or pancreatic fistula
	Infusion or ingestion:
	Carbonic anhydrase inhibitors
	  (acetazolamide [Diamox])
	Hyperalimentation
	HCl, NH4Cl
	TPN
	
	Other:
	Eucapnic ventilation (normalizing
	PaCO$_2$ to 40 following prolonged
	hyperventilation) (e.g., hyper-
	ventilation from severe asthma or
	mechanical ventilation)

Management of Metabolic Acidosis

Problem – ↓ pH
Goal – Normalization of pH by ↑ HCO_3 or ↓ acid *

* Treat the primary ABG disorder. Secondary changes (i.e., compensations) will usually correct themselves after the primary disorder is corrected (unless the body is unable).

Therapy

Correct	Compensate
Correct underlying problem (acute or chronic)	Mechanical ventilation (to assist those in danger of muscle fatigue from hyperventilation)
Monitor/correct intake/output and electrolyte balance	
HCO_3 administration *	

* HCO_3 therapy (controversial) when < 15 mEq/L; < 10 mEq/L is considered an emergency

Examples:
Lactic acidosis – O_2 therapy and correct underlying cause
DKA – Insulin administration

Ventilator Management of Metabolic Acidosis

Situation: ↓ $PaCO_2$ with Normal pH (Compensated Metabolic Acidosis)
Problem: Improper hyperventilating in the attempt to correct for metabolic acidosis.
Solution: Correct metabolic acidosis before attempting to correct $PaCO_2$.

Metabolic Alkalosis

Definition	$HCO_3 > 26$ mEq/L
Cause	↓ Acid or ↑ Base
Compensation	Hypoventilation

Overview of Parameter Changes

	pH	$PaCO_2$	HCO_3	K^+	Cl^-
Uncompensated*	↑	↑	↑	↓	↓
Partially Compensated (PC) (chronic)	↑	↑	↑	↓	↓
Full Compensated (FC) chronic**	N	↑	↑↑	N	N

* Rare. If there is no compensation, there is usually a secondary respiratory alkalosis. Hence there is usually no distinction between acute and chronic.

** This classification essentially does not exist because $PaCO_2$ generally does not return pH back to normal range (usually only ½ way back). If pH is normal, there is usually a secondary respiratory disorder at work.

Determining Compensation

Expected Change in pH and $PaCO_2$ for Every 1 mEq/L ↑ in HCO_3

	Expected ↑ in pH*	Expected ↑ in $PaCO_2$ (mmHg)**
Acute and Chronic	0.015	0.7-1.5 (max)

*   For ease of calculation, for every 1 mEq/L ↑ in HCO_3, the last digit of pH ↑ 1.5.

**   Compensation (expected $PaCO_2$) is highly variable – anywhere between 0.25 – 1.0 with 0.7 the average (see below). Maximal compensation is rare and limited (see below). When maximal compensation does occur, $PaCO_2$ = last two digits of pH

Equation

$$\text{Expected } PaCO_2 = [(0.7 \times HCO_3) + 21] \ (\pm 5)$$

Quick Reference Chart – Expected Values

↑ HCO₃	↑ pH*	↑ PaCO₂ (max) **
50	7.79	58 (79)
48	7.76	57 (76)
46	7.73	55 § (73)
44	7.70	54 (70)
42	7.67	53 (67)
40	7.64	51 (64)
38	7.61	50 (61)
36	7.58	48 (58)
34	7.55	47 § (55)
32	7.52	46 (52)
30	7.49	44 (49)
28	7.46	43 (46)
26	7.43	41 (43)
24	7.40	40

* From a normal pH of 7.40
** Maximal compensation: $PaCO_2$ = last two digits of pH
   Normal respiratory compensation is weak, variable, and rarely, if ever, full or maximum due to:
   1) The body's desire to maintain a normal pH/$PaCO_2$ and
   2) Hypoventilation often leads to hypoxemia which stimulates a hypoxic drive.

Therefore, compensated $PaCO_2$ is usually less than max (i.e., averages 0.7) and the pH usually only returns less than ½ of the way back towards normal, unless a very mild metabolic alkalosis exists.

§ It has been typically thought that hypoventilation rarely occurs above this level, yet it can and does occur.
Values of $PaCO_2$ higher than 55 mmHg more typically indicate a secondary respiratory acidosis.
Values of $PaCO_2$ less than expected may have a secondary respiratory alkalosis.

Signs & Symptoms of Metabolic Alkalosis

Hypoventilation (compensation)	Tingling / numbness	Seizures / Tetany Stupor
Lightheadedness	Tachycardia	Coma
Headache	Palpitations	Death
	Lethargy	

	Physiological Effects	Clinical Manifestations
Cardio-pulm. System	Bronchoconstriction ↑ myocardial irritability (early) ↓ myocardial contractility (late) Pulmonary vasodilation Systemic vasoconstriction	Hypoventilation Arrhythmias ↑ HR, palpitations ↓ PVR Pale skin color
CNS	Constricted cerebral vessels (↓ cerebral edema) ↑ excitability and NM irritab. ↑or ↓ respiratory center activity	↓ CSF pressure Anxiety, nervousness, light-headedness, tingling/numbness, ↓reflexes, lethargy, confusion, seizures, tetany, coma Hypoventilation (limited)
Renal & Metabol.	↓Serum Cl⁻ and K⁺ ↓ excretion of K⁺ Excretion of HCO₃	Hyper/hypochloremia Hypokalemia ↓ urine K⁺

Causes of Metabolic Alkalosis

↑ Base (HCO₃)	↓ Acid	
Intestinal intake: Antacid administration NaHCO₃ administration **↓ Cl⁻ (causes ↑ HCO₃):** Bartters syndrome Cushing's syndrome Diarrhea Hyperaldosteronism Severe ↓ K⁺	**↑ Kidney Excretion:** Chronic renal failure Diuretic therapy **(most common cause)** Hypokalemia (severe) Hypochloremia (severe) Hypovolemia (severe) **Intestinal loss:** Nasogastric suctioning Vomiting (severe)	**Drugs:** Diuretics Systemic steroids **Other:** Eucapnic ventilation (normalizing $PaCO_2$) of chronic CO_2 retainer (i.e., excessive MV)

Management of Metabolic Alkalosis

Problem – ↑ pH
Goal – Normalization of pH by ↓ HCO_3 or ↑ acid *

* Treat the primary ABG disorder. Secondary changes (i.e., compensations) will usually correct themselves after the primary disorder is corrected (unless the body is unable).

Therapy

Correct	Compensate*
Correct underlying problem (acute or chronic)	Acid infusion (HCl, NH_4Cl)
	Carbonic anhydrase inhibitor
Correct volume depletion	(acetazolamide [Diamox])
Replenish K^+, Cl^- and Mg^+ deficits	HCO_3 dialysis

* Specific and limited indications for persistent alkalosis

Ventilator Management of Metabolic Alkalosis

Situation: ↑ $PaCO_2$ with Normal pH (Compensated Metabolic Alkalosis)

Problem: Hypoventilating to correct for metabolic alkalosis.
Solution: Correct metabolic alkalosis first, otherwise increasing $\dot{V}E$ to
↓ $PaCO_2$ will worsen the metabolic alkalosis (further ↑ of pH)
potentially causing cardiac dysrhythmias, seizures, or other
neurological problems.

Mixed Metabolic Disorders

(AG Metab. acidosis PLUS Non-AG Met. acidosis +/or Met. alkalosis)
When there is an ↑ Anion Gap, if:

$\downarrow HCO_3 = \uparrow AG$	Then there is an AG Metab. Acidosis HCO_3 fall = AG rise Expected 1↓ in HCO_3 for each 1↑ in AG
$\downarrow\downarrow HCO_3 > \uparrow AG$	Then AG Metab. Acid. + Non AG Metab. Acidosis HCO_3 falls greater than the AG rise Lower HCO_3 than expected - Acid is being added
$\downarrow HCO_3 < \uparrow\uparrow AG$	Then AG Metab. Acid. + Metab. Alkalosis HCO_3 falls less than the AG rise More HCO_3 than expected - HCO_3 is being added

Examples:

Cations		
Na⁺ 140		
Normal Anions		
AG 12	HCO₃ 24	Cl⁻ 104
Pure Non-AG Acidosis (Hyperchloremic)		
AG 12	HCO₃ ↓20	Cl⁻ ↑108
Pure AG Acidosis		
AG ↑24	HCO₃ ↓12	Cl⁻ 104
AG Acidosis + Non AG Acidosis (Hyperchloremic)		
AG ↑24	HCO₃ ↓8	Cl⁻ ↑108
AG Acidosis + Metabolic Alkalosis		
AG ↑24	HCO₃ ↑16	Cl⁻ ↓100

Diagnosing Mixed Metabolic Disorders

Oakes Method
Bicarbonate Gap (BG)
(also commonly called Corrected HCO_3 or Delta Gap)

$$BG = Patient's\ HCO_3 + \Delta\ AG\ *$$

Normal = 24 † =	AG Metabolic Acidosis
< 20 =	AG Metabolic Acidosis + Non AG Metabolic Acidosis
> 28 =	AG Metabolic Acidosis + Metabolic Alkalosis

† Allow for ± 4 ($HCO_3 + \Delta\ AG$ = 20-28)

Examples

Pure Anion Gap	AG + Non AG	AG + Metab. Alkal.
HCO_3 16; AG 20	HCO_3 8; AG 20	HCO_3 22; AG 20
BG =16 + (20-12) = 24	BG =8 + (20-12) = 16	BG = 22 + (20-12) = 30
Diabetic (DKA)	Diabetic (DKA) with diarrhea	Cardiac arrest with $NaHCO_3$ admin.

Other Methods to Diagnose Mixed Metabolic Disorders

$\Delta\ AG : \Delta\ HCO_3$* (called Delta Ratio)
$\uparrow AG = \downarrow HCO_3$ (ratio 1)   = AG Metab. Acidosis
$\uparrow AG < \downarrow HCO_3$ (ratio < 1) = AG Metab Acid. + Non AG Metab Acid.
$\uparrow AG > \downarrow HCO_3$ (ratio > 2) = AG Metab. Acid. + Metab. Alkalosis

$\Delta\ AG - \Delta\ HCO_3$ (called Delta-Delta)
Normal = 0 = AG Metabolic Acidosis
< - 6 = AG Metabolic Acidosis + Non AG Metabolic Acidosis
> +6 = AG Metabolic Acidosis + Metabolic Alkalosis

*Note:
$\Delta\ AG$ = Delta Gap (measured AG – normal AG)
(i.e., patient's AG – 12)
$\Delta\ HCO_3$ = Delta HCO_3 (normal HCO_3 – measured HCO_3)
(i.e., 24 – patient's HCO_3.)

ABGs in COPD

Abnormal baselines in COPD patients may = Chronic Respiratory Acidosis (see pg 10). If so, these patient's are known as "CO_2 Retainers".

> **Typical abnormal baseline:**
> Low normal pH (7.35 – 7.39)
> ↑ $PaCO_2$ (typically > 50)
> ↑ HCO_3

Effects of Common Complications for a CO_2 Retainer

1) Acute Exacerbations

A) Acute Lung Infection

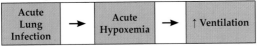

Result: Acute Respiratory Alkalosis superimposed on a baseline of Chronic Respiratory Acidosis (acute on chronic condition)

Example: pH 7.48, $PaCO_2$ 40, HCO_3 28, PaO_2 60
Technical Classification: Metabolic Alkalosis (Uncompensated)

Actual Interpretation:

Chronic Respiratory Acidosis + Acute Respiratory Alkalosis	
Baseline:	
pH 7.36	pH 7.48
$PaCO_2$ 54 →→→→	$PaCO_2$ 40
HCO_3 30	HCO_3 28
PaO_2 55	PaO_2 60

> **DANGER:** Treatment is much different for Respiratory Alkalosis than for Metabolic Alkalosis

B) Heart Failure

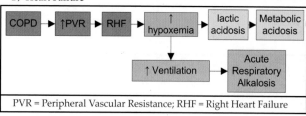

PVR = Peripheral Vascular Resistance; RHF = Right Heart Failure

Example: pH 7.41, PaCO$_2$ 36, HCO$_3$ 24, PaO$_2$ 44

Technical Classification: Normal ABG with hypoxemia !! (If on oxygen, then even PaO$_2$ may be within a normal range).

Actual Interpretation:

Chronic Resp Acidosis	+ Respiratory Alkalosis	+ Metabolic Acidosis
Baseline: pH 7.36 PaCO$_2$ 54 →→→→ HCO$_3$ 30 PaO$_2$ 55	pH 7.48 PaCO$_2$ 40 HCO$_3$ 28 →→→→ PaO$_2$ 49	pH 7.41 PaCO$_2$ 36 HCO$_3$ 24 PaO$_2$ 44

Patient history, ABG baseline, assessment and serial ABGs are essential.

Result: Acute Respiratory Alkalosis and Metabolic Acidosis superimposed on Chronic Respiratory Acidosis

2. Muscle Fatigue

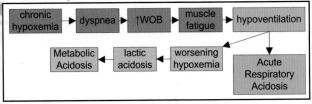

Example: pH 7.14, PaCO$_2$ 70, HCO$_3$ 28, PaO$_2$ 44

Technical Classification: Acute Respiratory Acidosis

Actual Interpretation:

Chronic Resp Acidosis	+ Acute Resp Acidosis	+ Metabolic Acidosis
pH 7.36	pH 7.20	pH 7.14
PaCO$_2$ 54→→→→	PaCO$_2$ 74	PaCO$_2$ 70
HCO$_3$ 30	HCO$_3$ 32 →→→→	HCO$_3$ 28
PaO$_2$ 55	PaO$_2$ 49	PaO$_2$ 44

Result: Acute Respiratory Acidosis and Metabolic Acidosis superimposed on Chronic Respiratory Acidosis

Therapy based on initial classification would be intubation and MV.
Correct therapy would be to first try and alleviate the hypoxemia and ↓ WOB
with a controlled trial of O$_2$ therapy. Apply NPPV, if needed.

3. Therapeutic Complications

A) Inappropriate Mechanical Ventilation

Ventilating these patients to a "normal" $PaCO_2$ of 40 mmHg will result in exactly the same effect as acute lung infection (above), an Acute Respiratory Alkalosis superimposed on Chronic Respiratory Acidosis. Do not normalize the $PaCO_2$ to 40. Proper ventilation should be geared towards normalizing the pH to the patient's baseline, not the $PaCO_2$.

Results of abruptly lowering the $PaCO_2$ and increasing the pH beyond their baseline may lead to ↓ cerebral blood flow (CBF), ↓ CO, arrhythmias, seizures, and difficulty weaning.

B) Drug Administration

Drugs common to COPD therapy (diuretics, systemic steroids) can all cause a concurrent Non-Anion Gap Metabolic Alkalosis (↑ HCO_3) resulting in a high "normal" pH (7.41 – 7.45).

C) Oxygen Therapy (*Hypoxic Drive Theory*)

For many years a common misconception has been propagated that "CO_2 retainers" (or, for that matter, all COPD patients) breathe on a hypoxic drive only and that the administration of oxygen therapy, to above hypoxemia levels, will "wipe out" the patient's drive to breathe. This, in turn, will lead to hypoventilation, resulting in an increased $PaCO_2$, decreased pH, and ventilatory failure!

Repeated studies have shown this myth to be without foundation.

A detailed explanation of why this myth is not true (and references) are available at www.RespiratoryUpdate.com.

Basic Points To Remember with O_2 Administration in Patients with COPD

A. Drive to Breathe

1. The more hypoxic a patient, the greater the hypoxic drive to breathe.
2. However, the hypoxic drive is normally only approximately 10% of the overall drive to breathe, *even in CO_2 retainers*.
3. CO_2 retainers are NOT dependent on the hypoxic drive to breathe and an increase in FIO_2 will never "wipe out" the $pH/PaCO_2$ drive to breathe (only the O_2 drive will be eliminated if $PaO_2 > 170$).
4. $pH/PaCO_2$ will usually always be the main drive to breathe, except in very severe hypoxia.
5. **For these reasons, keeping a CO_2 retainer hypoxemic in order to maintain their O_2 drive is NEVER justified and is clinically contraindicated.**

B. CO_2 Retention

1. An increase in FIO_2 in a stable CO_2 retainer may cause the $PaCO_2$ to rise slightly, but will usually have a clinically insignificant effect.
2. An increase in FIO_2 in a CO_2 retainer during an acute exacerbation may cause the $PaCO_2$ to rise due to reasons other than wiping out the O_2 drive to breathe (see www.RespiratoryUpdate.com), This rise in CO_2 may significantly contribute to the increase WOB and fatigue of the patient trying to blow off the excess CO_2, resulting in a further rise of $PaCO_2$ and drop in pH.
3. **HOWEVER, it is NEVER justified to keep a patient hypoxemic in order to prevent a rise in CO_2. Hypercarbia is easily managed with assisted ventilation (e.g., NIV) and the hypoxemia is easily managed with O_2 therapy.**

Oxygenation Assessment

Evaluating Oxygen Status

Oxygenation at the Lungs (external respiration)			Oxygenation at the Tissues (internal respiration)		
	Norm	Abnorm		Norm	Abnorm
Adequacy					
PaO_2	80-100 mmHg	< 80 mmHg	$P\bar{v}O_2$	35-42 mmHg	< 35 or > 45 mmHg
CaO_2	15-24 mL/dL	↑↓	$C\bar{v}O_2$	12-15 mL/dL	↑↓
SaO_2	> 95%	< 95%	$S\bar{v}O_2$	60-80%	< 60%
SpO_2	> 95%	< 95%	$Pa\text{-}vO_2$	60 mmHg	↑↓
			$Ca\text{-}\bar{v}O_2$	4.5-5.0 mL/dL	↑↓
Efficiency					
PAO_2	100 mmHg	< 90 mmHg	$O_{2_{ER}}$	25%	↑↓
$PA\text{-}aO_2$	10-25 mmHg (air) 30-50 mmHg (100%)	>25 mmHg	$\dot{V}O_2$	200-250 mL/min	↑↓
			$\dot{D}O_2$	750 - 1000 mL/min	↑↓
PaO_2/PAO_2	0.8-0.9	<0.6	VQI	0.8	↑↓
PaO_2/FIO_2	>300	<300			
$PA\text{-}aO_2/PaO_2$	<1.0	>1.0			
Q_S/Q_T phys	2-5%	> 20%			

Lung Adequacy

PaO_2 Assessment

Normal Value: 80 – 100 mm Hg

Normal Variations – Due to FIO_2, barometric pressure, or age
(PaO$_2 \approx 110 - \frac{1}{2}$ patient's age)

Abnormal Variations –
  Hyperoxemia = Above normal values
  Hypoxemia = Below normal values
            For Levels of Hypoxemia, see page 72

SaO_2/SpO_2 Assessment

SaO_2 = Calculated O_2 saturation from PaO_2 (if an analysis)
    (actual measured value if with a co-oximeter)
SpO_2 = Peripheral O_2 saturation (measured value of Hb saturation with a
    pulse oximeter).

Normal Value = 95 – 97%

PaO2-SaO2 Relationship

PaO_2	SaO_2*
150	100 %
100	97 %
80	95 %
60	90 %
55	88 %
40	75 %

*varies with shifts in
oxyhemoglobin curve

Note:
Always check for proper correlation between the PaO_2/SaO_2 calculated values and the measured SpO_2 value.

SEE ACCURACY CHECK, page 94

SaO_2/SpO_2 will NOT detect hyperoxemia

Factors affecting SaO_2 and/or SpO_2 readings - See AARC Clinical Practice Guideline, page 98

Oxyhemoglobin Dissociation Curve

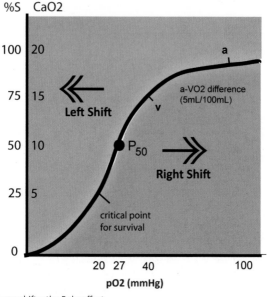

Curve shift = the Bohr effect

a = normal arterial blood; v = normal venous blood

P_{50} = PaO_2 @ 50% Saturation (normal = 27 mmHg)

Left Shift ↑ Hgb-O_2 affinity - ↓ P_{50}	Right Shift ↓ Hgb-O_2 affinity - ↑ P_{50}
Alkalosis	Acidosis
↓ Temp, ↓ PCO_2, ↓ PO^4, ↓ 2,3 DPG	↑ Temp, ↑ PCO_2, ↑ PO^4, ↑ 2,3 DPG
Polycythemia	Anemias (sickle cell)
Abnormal Hgb (fetal, CO, Met)	Chronic Hypoxemia (high altit.)

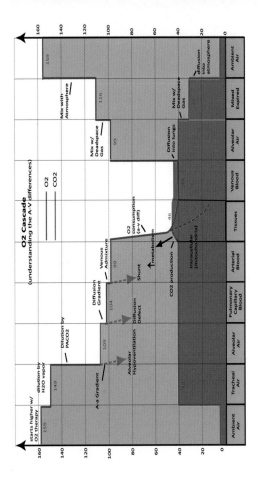

Oxygenation Assessment

Hypoxemia
Levels of Hypoxemia

	PaO$_2$	SpO$_2$ %	Clinical Notes	Hypoxia
Mild Hypoxemia	60-79 mmHg	90-94%		Unlikely
Moderate Hypoxemia	40-59 mmHg	75-89%		Unlikely if cardiovascular system able to compensate
Severe Hypoxemia	< 40 mmHg	< 75%	30: Loss of consciousness 20: Brain damage likely	Likely

Note: PaO$_2$ may give "false positive" results. The patient may have a good PaO$_2$, but still hypoxic.

Reason: Either ↓ CaO$_2$ or tissue can't metabolize the O$_2$.

Causes: anemia, ↓ cardiac output, carbon monoxide or cyanide poison, hypothermia, peripheral shunting, methemoglobinemia. See table page 73.

Refractory Hypoxemia: Hypoxemia that shows no or little ↑ PaO$_2$ with ↑ FIO$_2$.
   -- Defined as < 5 mmHg ↑ PaO$_2$ with 0.1 ↑ FIO$_2$.
Responsive Hypoxemia: Hypoxemia that shows a significant ↑ PaO$_2$ with
   ↑ FIO$_2$. Defined as > 5 mmHg ↑ PaO$_2$ with 0.1 ↑FIO$_2$.

Hypoxemic Respiratory Failure
Known as: Type I Acute Respiratory Failure (ARF), Lung Failure,
      Oxygenation Failure, or Respiratory Insufficiency
Definition: The failure of the lungs and heart to provide adequate
      O$_2$ to meet metabolic needs.
Criteria: PaO$_2$ < 60 mmHg on FIO$_2$ ≥ 0.50 -or-
      PaO$_2$ < 40 mmHg on any FIO$_2$ -and/or-
      SaO$_2$ < 90 %

Signs & Symptoms of Acute Hypoxemia/Hypoxia (Relative order of appearance)		Signs & Symptoms of Chronic Hypoxemia/Hypoxia
Tachypnea	Confusion	Arrhythmias
Dyspnea	Euphoria	↓ CO
Pallor	Bradycardia	Clubbing (sometimes)*
Tachycardia	Hypotension	Dyspnea
Hypertension	Nausea/vomiting	Irritability
Headache	Loss of coordination	Tiredness
Anxiety	Lethargy/weakness	Papilledema
Cyanosis	Tremors	Polycythemia
Arrhythmias	Hyper-active reflexes	Impaired judgment
Blurred or tunnel vision	Stupor	Myoclonic jerking
Impaired judgment	Coma ≈ 30 mmHg	Pulmonary hypertension
	Death	

* Only some diseases, such as bronchiectasis, cystic fibrosis, interstitial lung disease, and lung abscess.

Types and Causes of Hypoxemia and Hypoxia

Types	Causes	Examples
Atmospheric	Insufficient O_2 available	$\downarrow FIO_2$: Drowning (no FIO_2); O_2 therapy error ($\downarrow FIO_2 <$ 0.21), smoke inhalation $\downarrow PAO_2$: High altitude ($PaO_2 \downarrow 4$ mmHg/1000 ft)
Tidal	**Hypoventilation** ($\uparrow PaCO_2, \rightarrow \downarrow PaO_2$)	Many causes of pulmonary compromise
Alveolar	1. **Deadspace (alveolar)** (wasted ventilation; ventilation without perfusion) (Deadspace Unit; V/0) (Deadspace Effect; V/$\downarrow$Q) (see pages 40 & 41)	**↑ Alveolar deadspace :** a) Complete block: Pulmonary embolus (air, blood, fat, tumor) b) $\downarrow$ blood flow: Shock, cardiac arrest, $\uparrow$ PVR, air trap c) $\uparrow$V/$\downarrow$Q: $\uparrow$ MV and/or PEEP ($\uparrow$ lung zones 1+2 from $\uparrow$ Palv)
	2. **Shunt** A) **Absolute (True) Shunt**** (Perfusion without ventilation; 0/Q) B) **Relative shunt** (perfusion with $\downarrow$ventilation; $\downarrow$V/Q) (V/Q mismatch, shunt effect, or venous admixture)	**Anatomical shunts:** Pleural, bronchial, thebesian veins, anatomical defects **Capillary shunts +/or Shunt effect:** a) Alveoli collapsed, fluid filled or blocked (complete or partial): ARDS, atelectasis (most common), cystic fibrosis, pneumonia, pneumothorax, pulmonary edema b) $\downarrow$ or no alveolar ventilation: Airway obstruction, asthma, COPD, position changes, secretions, etc.
	3. **Diffusion Defect** ($\uparrow$ a-c membrane thickness)	Fibrosis, Proteinosis, Sarcoidosis

Types	Causes	Examples
Hemoglobic*	Blood abnormality ($\downarrow CaO_2$)	Anemia, hemorrhage, sickle cell, CO poison Shift of oxyhemoglobin dissociation curve to right
Stagnant*	Blood perfusion abnormality ($\downarrow O_2$ transport)	CV failure, arrythmias, hemorrhage, shock
Histotoxic §	Tissue can't metabolize O_2	Cyanide or ethanol poisoning
Demand	$\uparrow$ Metabolic demand for more O_2 (which then causes one or more of the above hypoxemic conditions)	Burns, exercise, fever, hyperthyroidism, sepsis

* Hypoxemia may or may not be present with hypoxia

** O_2 therapy is usually ineffective in absolute shunts (refractory hypoxemia) because the O_2 can't get to the blood. In capillary shunts, rarely is the problem purely absolute, there is usually some relative shunting as well.

§ Rarely accompanied by hypoxemia

MIX & MATCH: Very often, disease processes produce more than one type of hypoxemia!
e.g., COPD (alveolar from V/Q mismatch and stagnant from cor pulmonale)
Smoke inhalation (atmospheric from $\downarrow O_2$ in room, alveolar from airway constriction, hemoglobic from CO poisoning, histotoxic from cyanide poisoning)
Premature babies (alveolar from surfactant deficiency, stagnant from persistent fetal circulation, and hemoglobic from fetal Hb)

Oxygenation Assessment

Distinguishing Types of Hypoxemia

Types	PAO_2	PaO_2	$PA\text{-}aO_2$	$Pa\text{-}vO_2$	$PaCO_2$	$PACO_2$	$Pa\text{-}ACO_2$
Atmospheric	↓	↓	N	N	↓	↓	N
Tidal	↓	↓	N↑	N	↑	↑	N
Alveolar							
Deadspace	N↓	N↓	N↕	N↕	N↕	↓	↑
Absolute Shunt	N↑	↓	↑	N	N↕	N↕	N↕
V/Q Mismatch (relative shunt)	N	↓	↑	N	N↕	N↕	N↕
Diffusion defect	N	N↓	↑	N	N↓	N↓	N
Hemoglobic	N	N	N	N	N↓	N↓	N
Stagnant	N	↓	↑	↑↑	N↕	N↕	N↕
Histotoxic	N	N	N	↓	N	N	N
Demand	*Any of the above*						

PAO_2 = Alveolar Air Equation

$PAO_2 = ([PB - PH2O] \times FIO_2) - PaCO_2\,(1.25)$
$\quad\quad\quad = PIO_2 - PaCO_2\,(1.25)$
$\quad\quad\quad = 150 - PaCO_2\,(1.25)$ on room air

Normal = 100 mmHg (room air)
$\quad\quad\quad\;\; = 663$ mmHg (100%, sea level)

Estimate = $(FIO_2 \times 700) - 50$

A-a Gradient ($PA\text{-}aO_2$)

1) $PAO_2 - PaO_2$ (Alveolar air equation – ABG value)
2) $150 - (PaO_2 + [PaCO_2 \times 1.25])$ (150 – ABG values) (room air only)

Hypoxemia Diagnostic Algorithm

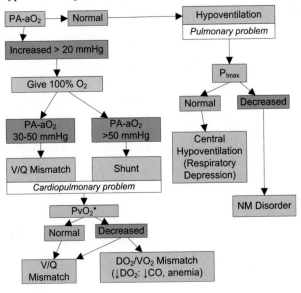

CO = Cardiac Output

* PvO_2 is obtained from a CVP line or PA catheter

Lung Efficiency
Estimating Degree of Pulmonary Dysfunction

Index	Normal	Abnormals
a/A Ratio (PaO_2 / PAO_2)	0.8 – 0.9 (any FIO_2) (0.75 elderly)	< 0.6 = shunt, V/Q mismatch, diffusion defect < 0.35 = indicative of weaning failure (?) < 0.15 = refractory hypoxemia
$PA\text{-}aO_2$ (A-a Gradient; A-aDO2) $[PAO_2 - PaO_2]$	10 – 25 mmHg (room air) (↑ with age up to 35) 30 – 50 mmHg (100% O_2)	> 25 mmHg (> 35 with age) (21% O_2) *Estimate = 0.3 x age* > 30 – 50 mmHg (100% O_2) > 350 is often indicative of weaning failure
P/F Ratio (PaO_2 / FIO_2)	400 – 500 (regardless of FIO_2)	300 – 400 = mod. pulmonary dysfun. 200 – 300 = acute lung injury (ALI) < 200 = ARDS
$\dfrac{PA\text{-}aO_2}{PaO_2}$ (Respiratory Index; RI)	< 1.0	> 1.0 > 5.0 = refractory hypoxemia
Shunt	2-5% (< 10%)	See estimating shunt below

Notes:

a/A Ratio

More stable with FIO_2 changes than A-a Gradient: A-a gradient changes with FIO_2, a/A remains stable. Changes only with $PaCO_2$ and V/Q changes.

Can be used to calculate desired PaO_2 and FIO_2 (See page 87)

$PA\text{-}aO_2$

Varies with age and FIO_2.

Can be used to estimate shunt (see next page), and can be used to distinguish between true shunt, V/Q mismatch, and diffusion defect (See page 79)

Increases = ↑ shunt, V/Q mismatch, hypoventilation, or ↓ diffusion.

Estimate: $PA\text{-}aO_2 = 140 - (PaO_2 + PaCO_2)$ (on 21% only)   or

$\qquad = 150 - (PaO_2 + [PaCO_2 \times 1.25])$ (on 21% only)

P/F Ratio

Can be used to calculate desired PaO_2 and FIO_2 (See page 88)

See PaO_2/FIO_2 relationship on page 87

Can be used to estimate shunt (see next page)

Oxygenation Ratio = when FIO2 is used as a % (i.e, PaO_2/FIO_2%)

Estimating Shunt (Q_S/Q_T)

1) PaO_2

Q_S/Q_T = 5% additional shunt (added to normal 5%) for every 100 mmHg PaO_2 is below expected. Most accurate on 100% O_2. (See page 87)

2) PaO_2 / FIO_2 (P/F Ratio)

PaO_2/FIO_2	% Shunt	Clinical Significance
> 400	≤ 5%	Normal
300-400	5-15%	Moderate pulmonary dysfunction
200-300	15-20%	Acute Lung Injury (Mild ARDS)
< 200	> 20%	ARDS (Mod-Sev ARDS)

3) PA-aO_2

$Q_S/QT = PA$-$aO_2 / 20$

Most accurate when breathing 100% O_2, but 50% O_2 x 15-20 minutes is preferred due to ↑ shunting from absorption atelectasis.

PA-aO_2: Distinguishing Shunts and Diffusion Defects

	Room Air	100% O_2 **
No Shunting	Normal PA-aO_2 < 25 *	Normal PA-aO_2 30-50
Absolute Shunt	↑ PA-aO_2 > 25	↑ PA-aO_2 > 50
V/Q Mismatch	↑ PA-aO_2 > 25	Normal PA-aO_2 30-50
Diffusion Defect	PA-aO_2 same	

* Normal PA-aO_2 may ↑ up to 35 with advanced age.
** In clinical practice, administration of 100% O_2 for 20 minutes will worsen the shunt due to absorption atelectasis. Therefore, 50% O_2 is given to see if PaO_2 > 150 (normal) or < 150 (shunting).

Assessment of Tissue Oxygenation (ABC)

Supply
A. Arterial/Venous O_2 Assessment   (See Oxygenation Assessment – page 68)

Delivery

B. Blood Hemoglobin Assessment   male 13-18 gm/dl or g%
 female 12-16 gm/dl or g%
 	
 Anemia
    Mild anemia: 10-12 g% - hypoxia unlikely due to ↑ CO
    Moderate anemia: 6-9 g% - hypoxia may occur
    Severe anemia: < 6 g% - hypoxia is likely
   Cyanosis (> 5 gm reduced Hb; acrocyanosis, central)
   Polycythemia

C. Cardiovascular Assessment	3) Blood volume
1) Heart	a. Urinary output
a. Cardiac output (4-8 L/min)	b. CVP (0-6 mmHg)
Cardiac index (2.5-4.4 L/min/m²)	c. Skin turgor
Heart rate (60-100 beats/min)	
Stroke volume (60-120 mL/beat)	4) Combined
b. Arrhythmias	a. BP (120/80)
2) Vessels	b. Capillary refill (< 3 sec)
a. Vascular tone	c. Edema (pitting scale)
1. SVR	d. Pulse
2. PVR	

O_2 **Content**

$$CaO_2 = (Hg \times 1.36) \times SaO_2 + (PaO_2 \times 0.0031)$$

A-a Gradient (PA-aO₂) (A-aDO₂) Alveolar- arterial O₂ tension difference	Normal = 10 - 25 mm Hg (air) = 30 - 50mm Hg (100% O₂) Increases with age and FIO₂. PaO₂ is calculated at FIO₂ 0.5 breathed x 20 min to get PaO₂ > 150 (100% not used due to ↑ shunt).	Indicates efficiency of gas exchange. Normal values =normal shunt. Distinguishes between true shunt and V/Q mismatch. ↑ = shunt, V/Q mismatch, alveolar hypoventilation, or ↓ diffusion. > 350 mmHg indicative of weaning failure. Less accurate estimate (on 21% only).
1) $PA\text{-}aO_2 = PAO_2 - PaO_2$		
2) $PA\text{-}aO_2 = 140 - (PaO_2 + PaCO_2)$	ABG is drawn for $PaCO_2$ and PaO_2.	See shunt equation.
3) $PA\text{-}aO_2 / 20$	Estimate of shunt (100% O_2)	
Alveolar O₂ Tension (Alveolar air equation) (PAO₂)	Normal =100 mm Hg(air) = 663 mm Hg (100%, sea level) RE = respiratory exchange ratio (normal = 0.8)	Partial pressure of O₂ in alveoli. Used to determine alveolar O₂ tension to calculate PA-aO₂ gradient, a/A ratio, and % shunt.
1) $PaO_2 = ([PB - PH_2O] \times FIO_2) - PaCO_2 \times (FIO_2 + 1 - FIO_2/RE)$	Short form when breathing < 100% O_2	
2) $PaO_2 = ([PB - PH_2O] \times FIO_2) - PaCO_2 (1.25)$	Short form when breathing 100% O_2, $PIO_2 = (PB - PH_2O) \times FIO_2$ Estimate only on room air	
3) $PaO_2 = PIO_2 - PaCO_2 (1.25)$	Estimate only	
4) $PaO_2 = 150 - PaCO_2 (1.25)$		
5) $PaO_2 = (FIO_2 \times 700) - 50$		

Arterial/Alveolar O₂ Tension (a/A Ratio) PaO_2 / PAO_2 **PaO_2 known / PAO_2 calculated =** PaO_2 desired / PAO_2 unknown	Index of gas exchange function or efficiency of the lungs. Normal = 0.8 - 0.9 (0.75 elderly) at any FIO_2. Useful to predict PaO_2 when changing FIO_2 (See FIO_2 estimation equation)	More stable than A-a gradient: A-a gradient changes with FIO_2, a/A remains relatively stable with FIO_2 changes. Changes only with $PaCO2$ or V/Q changes. Low a/A (<0.6) = shunt, V/Q mismatch, or diffusion defect; < 0.35 = indicative of weaning failure, <0.15 = refractory hypoxemia. Can be used to estimate shunt (See shunt equation).
Arterial-(mixed)Venous O₂ Content Difference (Ca-$\bar{v}O_2$) $CaO_2 - C\bar{v}O_2 = Ca-\bar{v}O_2$	Difference between arterial and mixed venous O₂ contents. Normal = 4.2 - 5.0 mL/dL (vol%)	Represents O₂ consumption by tissue and estimate of cardiac output. ↑ = ↓CO or ↑ metabolism. ↓ = ↑CO or ↓ metabolism.
Arterial-(mixed)Venous O₂ Tension Difference (Pa-$\bar{v}O_2$ or a-$\bar{v}DO_2$) $PaO_2 - P\bar{v}O_2 = Pa-\bar{v}O_2$	Normal = 60 mm Hg	Difference between arterial and mixed venous O₂ tensions.
Arterial CO₂ tension ($PaCO_2$) $PaCO_2 = \dfrac{\dot{V}CO_2}{\dot{V}A}$	Normal = 35-45 mm Hg	

FIO2: Estimation 1) Using a/A ratio: $PAO_2 = PaO_2$ desired / a/A ratio 2) Using alveolar O_2 tension: $FIO_2 = PAO_2 + (PaCO_2 / 0.8) / (PB-H_2O)$ 3) Using A-a gradient: $FIO_2 = PA-aO_2 +$ desired $PaO_2 / 760$ 4) Using P/F Ratio: PaO_2 should be: $\dfrac{5\ PaO_2}{1\ FIO_2}$ 5) Estimate: $FIO_2 = PaO_2 / 500$	Figured at any FIO_2. Need ↑ FIO_2 x 20 minutes	Used to estimate the FIO_2 needed to achieve a desired PaO_2 or the PaO_2 that will be achieved at any given FIO_2, $\dfrac{\text{Current } PaO_2}{\text{Current } FIO_2} = \dfrac{\text{Desired } PaO_2}{\text{New } FIO_2}$ New $FIO_2 = PaO_2$ desired + $PaCO_2$ desired / (PaO_2 / PAO_2) / (PB - H_2O)
O_2 Consumption (Demand) ($\dot{V}O_2$) $\dot{V}O_2 = CO \times (CaO_2 - C\bar{v}O_2) \times 10$ $= CO \times Ca\text{-}\bar{v}O_2 \times 10$	Normal = 200 - 250 mL/min	Volume of O_2 consumed (utilized) by the body tissues per min. Index of metabolic level and CO. ↑$\dot{V}O_2$ = ↑metabolism or CO; ↓$\dot{V}O_2$ = ↓metabolism or CO
O_2 Consumption Index ($\dot{V}O_2 I$) $\dot{V}O_2 I = CI \times Ca\text{-}\bar{v}O_2 \times 10$	$\dot{V}O_2 I = \dot{V}O_2 / BSA$ = 110-165 mL/min/m²	O_2 consumption per body size.

O₂ Content (O_2 Content) 1) Arterial $CaO_2 = (Hgb \times 1.36) \times SaO_2 + (PaO_2 \times 0.0031)$ 2) Venous (mixed) $C\overline{v}O_2 = (Hgb \times 1.36) \times S\overline{v}O_2 + (P\overline{v}O_2 \times 0.0031)$ $= \dot{V}O_2/CO$ 3) Pulmonary capillary CcO_2	Normal = 15–24 mL/dL (vol%) Both 1.36 and 1.39 are considered correct. Hgb = gm % Normal = 12–15 mL/dL (vol%) $P\overline{v}O_2$ = pressure in mixed venous blood obtained from pulmonary artery. See shunt equation.	Total amount of O_2 in arterial blood (combined plus dissolved). Total amount of O_2 in mixed venous blood (combined plus dissolved). SaO_2 and $S\overline{v}O_2$ obtained from oximeter or oxyheme dissociation curve.
O₂ Delivery (Supply, Transport) ($\dot{D}O_2$) $\dot{D}O_2 = CO \times CaO_2 \times 10$	Normal = 750–1000 mL/min Quantity of O_2 delivered to the body tissues per minute. Requires CO determination.	$\uparrow O_2$ transport = $\uparrow CO$ +/or $\uparrow CaO_2$ $\downarrow O_2$ transport = $\downarrow CO$ +/or $\downarrow CaO_2$ 10 = conversion factor to mL/min
O₂ Delivery Index ($\dot{D}O_2 I$) $\dot{D}O_2 I = CI \times CaO_2 \times 10$	$\dot{D}O_2 I = \dot{D}O_2 / BSA$ $= 500$–600 mL/min/m²	O_2 delivery per body size.
O₂ Extraction Ratio (O_2 ER) O_2 ER = $\dfrac{O_2 \text{ consumption (demand)}}{O_2 \text{ delivery (supply)}}$ $= \dfrac{\dot{V}O_2}{\dot{D}O_2} \times 100$ $= \dfrac{Ca\text{-}\overline{v}O_2}{CaO_2}$	Normal = 25% Amount of O_2 extracted and consumed by the body tissues, relative to the amount delivered. Estimate = $\dfrac{Sa\text{-}\overline{v}O_2}{SaO_2}$	Indicator of O_2 supply/demand balance. $\uparrow$ratio = $\downarrow FO_2$ +/or $\uparrow O_2$ transport $\downarrow$ratio = $\uparrow O_2$ +/or $\downarrow O_2$ transport

Parameter	Formula	Normal / Values	Interpretation
O$_2$ Index (OI)	$OI = (\bar{P}aw \times FIO_2 \times 100) / PaO_2$		>40 = severe respiratory distress with high mortality; 20 - 25 = mortality > 50%
O$_2$ Reserve $O_2\ Reserve = \dot{D}O_2 - \dot{V}O_2$		Normal = 750 mL/min $= CO \times C\bar{v}O_2 \times 10$	Venous O$_2$ supply: O$_2$ supply minus O$_2$ demand
O$_2$ Saturation (mixed venous) (S$\bar{v}$O$_2$) $S\bar{v}O_2 = SaO_2 - \dot{V}O_2/\dot{D}O_2$ $= SaO_2 - Sa\text{-}\bar{v}O_2$		Normal = 75 % (60-80 %)	Percent of hemoglobin in mixed venous blood, saturated with O$_2$.
P/F Ratio (Oxygenation Ratio) PaO_2 / FIO_2		Normal = 400 – 500 (regardless of FIO$_2$) What PaO$_2$ Should Be: $\dfrac{5\ PaO_2}{1\ FIO_2\%}$	< 300 indicative of ALI < 200 = ARDS
Predicted PaO$_2$ (based on age)		$PaO_2 = 110 - \tfrac{1}{2}\ age$	
Respiratory Index (RI) $PA\text{-}aO_2 / PaO_2$		Normal = < 1.0	1.0 - 5.0 = V/Q mismatch > 5.0 = refractory hypoxemia due to physiol. shunt
Respiratory Quotient (Exchange ratio) (RQ, RE, RR) 1) $RQ = \dfrac{\dot{V}CO_2}{\dot{V}O_2}$ 2) $RQ = \dot{V}E \times \dfrac{F\bar{E}\ CO_2 - F_ICO_2}{F_IO_2 - F\bar{E}\ O_2}$ 3) $RQ = \dfrac{F\bar{E}\ CO_2}{FIO2 - F\bar{E}\ O_2}$		$\dfrac{\text{Volume } CO_2 \text{ produced/min}}{\text{Volume } O_2 \text{ consumed/min}}$ Normal = 200 / 250 = 0.8	RQ = ratio of CO$_2$ produced to O$_2$ consumed (internal respiration). RE represents the amount of O$_2$/CO$_2$ exchange in the lungs per minute (external respiration). RE = RQ in steady state condit.

Management of Oxygenation

Problem – ↓ PaO_2 and/or SaO_2
Goal – Prevent tissue hypoxia

Therapy

Correct	Compensate *
Correct underlying problem (acute or chronic)	O_2 therapy

* O_2 therapy is always done first and immediately to compensate the body while the underlying problem is addressed.

See AARC Evidence-Based Guideline *"Oxygen Therapy for Adults in the Acute Care Facility"*, page 97

Targets for Improving (Correcting) Oxygenation *

	PaO_2	SaO_2/SpO_2
Normal lung	≥ 80	≥95%
Mild lung injury	≥70	≥93%
Moderate lung injury	≥60	≥90%
Severe lung injury**	≥55	≥88%

* Permissive hypoxemia is gaining interest/acceptance when there is concern for O_2 toxicity and/or VILI (Ventilator Induced Lung Injury)
** In shunts > 50%, ↑ FIO_2 has little to no effect. Therefore, in these situations (e.g., ARDS) FIO_2 can be lowered to < 50% O_2 to reduce O_2 toxicity to the lungs without compromising PaO_2.

PaO_2/FIO_2 Relationship

What PaO_2 Should Be: $\dfrac{5\ PaO_2}{1\ FIO_2\ \%}$

$PaO_2 = 5 \times FIO_2\ \%$	= GOOD	(Perfect lungs)
$PaO_2 = 4 \times FIO_2\ \%$	= OK	(Low normal lungs)
$PaO_2 = 3 \times FIO_2\ \%$	= POOR	(Moderate lung dysfunction)
$PaO_2 = 2 \times FIO_2\ \%$	= BAD	(Severe lung dysfunction)

5/1 = Perfect lungs (PaO_2 will ↑ 5 mmHg for every 1% ↑ in FIO_2)
4/1 = Low normal (PaO_2 will ↑ 4 mmHg for every 1% ↑ in FIO_2)
3/1 = Typical COPD (PaO_2 will ↑ 3 mmHg for every 1% ↑ in FIO_2)
2/1 = Typical ARDS (PaO_2 will ↑ 2 mmHg for every 1% ↑ in FIO_2)

Responsive hypoxemia: PaO_2 will ↑ 5- 50 mmHg for every 10% ↑.
Refractory hypoxemia: PaO_2 will Δ < 5 mmHg for every 10% ↑.

Estimating $PaO_2/FIO_2\%$ Relationship

	Normal Lungs		Moderate Lung Dysfunction	Severe Lung Dysfunction
	5/1	4/1	3/1	2/1
FIO_2	PaO_2			
0.21	100	80	60	40
0.30	150	120	90	60
0.40	200	160	120	80
0.50	250	200	150	100
0.60	300	240	180	120
0.70	350	280	210	140
0.80	400	320	240	160
0.90	450	360	270	180
1.00	500	400	300	200

Calculating Desired PaO_2 and FIO_2

P/F Ratio (PaO_2 / FIO_2)	
$\dfrac{\text{Patient's } PaO_2}{\text{Patient's } FIO_2} = \dfrac{\text{Desired } PaO_2}{\text{Desired } FIO_2}$ or $\text{Desired } FIO_2 = \dfrac{\text{Desired } PaO_2 \times \text{Patient's } FIO_2}{\text{Patient's } PaO_2}$	Example: PaO_2 40 mmHg on room air $\dfrac{40}{0.21} = \dfrac{90}{x}$ $40x = 90 \times 0.21$ $x = \dfrac{90 \times 0.21}{40}$ $x = 0.47$ Desired $FIO_2 = 0.47$

a/A Ratio (PaO_2 / PAO_2)	
$\dfrac{\text{Patient's } PaO_2}{\text{Patient's } PAO_2} = \dfrac{\text{Desired } PaO_2}{\text{Desired } PAO_2}$ or $\text{Desired } PAO_2 = \dfrac{\text{Desired } PaO_2 \times \text{Patient's } PAO_2}{\text{Patient's } PaO_2}$	Example: PaO_2 40 mmHg on room air $\dfrac{40}{100} = \dfrac{90}{x}$ $40x = 90 \times 100$ $x = \dfrac{90 \times 100}{40}$ $x = 225$ Desired $PAO_2 = 225$

aO₂ / PaCO₂ Relationship

Remember Alveolar Air Equation:

$$P_AO_2 = 150 - (PaCO_2 \times 1.25) \text{ (on room air)}$$
$$P_aO_2 = 140 - (PaCO_2 \times 1.25) \text{ (assuming a normal shunt of 10 mmHg)}$$

$$PaO_2 + (PaCO_2 + ¼ PaCO_2) = 140$$

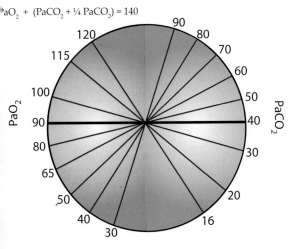

Note:

Values are approximate, on room air, and assume a normal shunt. PaO_2
  will be less at each level as shunt increases.

$PaO_2 < 30$: hypoxic death ensues

Therefore, a $PaCO_2 > 90$ is incompatible with life unless supplemental O_2
  is given.

$PaCO_2 \approx 16$: normal limit of hyperventilation

Oxygenation Assessment   89

Adjusted PaO$_2$

Adjusted PaO$_2$ = Actual PaO$_2$ without the influence of hyper or hypoventilation

$$= PaO_2 \pm (\Delta PaCO_2 \times 1.25)$$
Add value (+) if PaCO$_2$ is above 40
Subtract value (-) if PaCO$_2$ is lower than 40.

Primary Purpose: To determine proper O$_2$ management

Examples:

Determine the actual PaO$_2$, if PaCO$_2$ were 40.

Example 1	Example 2
Patient with PaCO$_2$ 60, PaO$_2$ 65. Does this patient need O$_2$ therapy?	Patient with PaCO$_2$ 30, PaO$_2$ 103. Does this patient need their O$_2$ therapy reduced?
Adjusted PaO$_2$ = Actual PaO$_2$ + (Δ PaCO$_2$ x 1.25) = 65 + (20 x 1.25) = 65 + 25 = 90	Adjusted PaO$_2$ = Actual PaO$_2$ − (Δ PaCO$_2$ x 1.25) = 103 − (10 x 1.25) = 103 − 13 = 90
The hypoxemia is due to hypoventilation and not a lung problem (i.e., shunting)	The hyperoxemia is due to hyperventilation and not O$_2$ administration
Ventilation therapy, not O$_2$ therapy is needed	O$_2$ therapy should not be reduced.

O$_2$ Therapy of Mechanically Ventilated Patients

Checklist for Worsening Oxygenation in Mechanically Ventilated Patients

Causes	Primary Strategies to Improve O$_2$ *
Patient:	Antibiotics
Airway obstruction / secretions	Bronchodilators
Anemia	Bronchoscopy
Artificial airway problem	CPAP/PEEP
Aspiration	CPT
Atelectasis	Diuretics
Bronchospasm	ET tube (suction, correct malposi-
Organ failure	tion, kinking, cuff, etc.)
Pneumonia	↑ FIO$_2$, $\overline{P}$aw, PEEP, TI, IRV
Pneumothorax	Fluids, vasopressors, inotropics
Pulmonary edema/emboli	Position changes (prone or continu-
Progression of underlying disease	ous lateral rotation)
Sepsis	Restore Hb level (>10 gm/100mL)
Shock	Thoracentesis / chest tube
Ventilator:	
Improper mode	Select appropriate mode
Improper settings (FIO$_2$, PEEP, V$_T$, etc.)	Correct settings
Leaks or disconnections	Find and fix
Malfunctions	Correct
Patient – ventilator asynchrony	Correct

* First correct primary cause, then adjust ventilator parameters (FIO$_2$, $\overline{P}$aw, PEEP, TI, modes) as needed.

Unconventional methods (ECMO, HFV, hyperbaric, intravascular oxygenation, etc.) may be employed when refractory hypoxemia (PaO$_2$ < 60 mmHg on FIO$_2$ ≥ 0.6) is not responsive to conventional MV and PEEP.

Improving Oxygenation (Correcting / Adjusting PaO_2 and SaO_2)

Goal: To maintain adequate O_2 delivery to the tissues while ventilating with the lowest possible FIO_2 and pressures.

Principle: PaO_2 is affected primarily by FIO_2, $\overline{Paw}$ (V_T, PIP, PEEP, T_I, $\dot{V}_I$, $\dot{V}_I$ waveform) and cardiovascular disease (i.e., optimizing lung volume and V/Q matching).
Adequate O_2 delivery to tissues is dependent on FIO_2, CO, and CaO_2.

Conventional Methods of Improving Oxygenation *

FIO_2	Keep FIO_2 as low as possible (< 0.5) to maintain PaO_2 60–100 mm Hg and/or SaO_2 > 90%. Note: When required, FIO_2 > 0.5 is preferred over high Palv. FIO_2 (required) = PaO_2 (desired) x FIO_2 (known) / PaO_2 (known)
PEEP/ CPAP	The adjustment of PEEP or CPAP is a key determinant of oxygenation, primarily due to the effect on $\overline{Paw}$. *See Indications next page*
$\overline{Paw}$	$\overline{Paw}$ is an important determinant of oxygenation. $PaO_2 \approx \overline{Paw}$ (until over-distension occurs, i.e., > upper inflection point on volume – pressure curve). ↑ $\overline{Paw}$ is indicated for patients with ↓ lung volume and refractory hypoxemia that does not respond to ↑ FIO_2 (e.g., ARDS). *Refractory hypoxemia* = PaO_2 < 60 mm Hg on $FIO_2 \geq 0.6$
IRV	**Purpose:** Increasing TI to ↑$\overline{Paw}$ and recruit and keep alveoli open for extended periods in order to improve V/Q, without over-inflating normal alveolar units. **Indication:** When conventional ventilator strategies with optimal PEEP have resulted in Pplat > 30 cm H_2O, without providing acceptable PaO_2/FIO_2 values. Use is controversial - consider specialty forms of IRV like APRV (BiVent)
Patient Positioning	Highly variable depending on disease type and patient status. Position changes effect: 1. Heart: venous return/cardiac output 2. Lungs: FRC/airway closure, diaph. displacement (COPD, obesity) 3. Heart/Lungs: V/Q distribution due to gravity and MV

* For unconventional methods of improving oxygenation, see Oakes' *Ventilator Management Pocket Guide*

Clinical	Physiological
Counteract auto-PEEP ↓ LV preload (cardiogenic pulmonary edema) Hypoxemia with FIO_2 > 0.5 Maintenance of collapsing alveoli (ARDS, postop atelectasis) Presence of artificial airway Stabilize chest wall (chest trauma)	PaO_2 < 60 mm Hg on FIO_2 0.5 PaO_2 ↑ < 10 mm Hg with FIO_2 ↑ of 0.2 $PA\text{-}aO_2$ > 300 on FIO_2 1.0 PaO_2/FIO_2 < 300

Clinical Note: CPAP indication is similar to PEEP. The primary difference is that CPAP requires the patient to do all the WOB. CPAP is appropriate if patient can spontaneously maintain a normal $PaCO_2$ without much difficulty and has been shown effective in limited applications to patients with hypoxemic respiratory failure. Typically, patients are not on CPAP alone for long periods of time. PS is usually added for patient comfort and decrease WOB.

* For a detailed coverage of the Commonly used Parameters for Measuring and Monitoring PEEP, Contraindications, Beneficial Effects, Potential Adverse Effects, Initiation of, PEEP Ranges, Determining Optimal PEEP, Using Applied PEEP in the presence of Auto-PEEP, Weaning from PEEP, and the PEEP/FIO_2 Algorithm of the ARDS Network, see Oakes' *Ventilator Management Pocket Guide*

ABG Accuracy Check (Checking for Errors)

1. **Check Patient – Does ABG line up with patient's clinical condition?**
   Good gases & patient distress; Bad gases & no patient distress?
   Rising or normal $PaCO_2$ in severe respiratory distress (e.g., asthma)

2. **Check Lab Values**
   HCO_3 should be within 1-2 mEq/L of Total CO_2 (electrolyte)
   (A difference of > 4 mEq/L = technical error)
   Actual HCO_3 should = 24 x $PaCO_2$/ (80 - last two digits of pH)
   (only works for pH between 7.30 – 7.50)

3. **Check for Errors**
   A) Sampling Errors
   1) Venous blood or contamination with venous blood
      ($\downarrow PaO_2$, $\uparrow PaCO_2$, $\uparrow$ pH). Venous $PaO_2 \approx 40$ (or does not match
      patient clinical condition; cross check with SpO_2).
   2) Air in sample - Effect varies with agitation, duration, temperature, & volume.
      PaO_2 higher than expected; $PaCO_2$ lower than expected.

Air	Blood
O_2 159 mmHg →	$\uparrow PaO_2$ (unless > 159)
CO_2 0 mmHg →	→ $PaCO_2$ →$\uparrow$ pH

   This can result in a negative $PA-aO_2$!

   Note: Samples drawn with a plastic syringe should never be
   placed in ice or in ice slush and should be analyzed within 30
   min. Samples to be analyzed > 30 min should be drawn in a
   glass syringe and placed in ice.
   3) Anticoagulant (heparin) - too much in sample (rare today, but
      same effect as air in sample).
   4) Patient not on reported FIO_2.
   5) Patient not in a steady state (sample taken too soon after a
      change in FIO_2 or MV).
   B) Measuring Errors
   1) Improper calibration, quality control, or sample mixing
   2) Documentation/Transcription errors
      ($PaCO_2 – PaO_2$ reversed? Orally conveyed?)
   3) Wrong patient blood

4) Time delay in measuring
    1. > 30 minutes un-iced (See above)
    2. > 60 minutes iced
5) ↑ WBC or platelets →↓ PaO_2 (leukocyte larceny)

4. Check PaO_2 – FIO_2 Relationship
    A) On Room Air: PaO_2 should be < 130 mmHg
    B) On ↑ FIO_2: PaO_2 should be < 5 x FIO_2
        Example: PaO_2 300 on 0.4 FIO_2 = error.
        Either PaO_2 is wrong or patient not on 0.4 FIO_2.
        (PaO_2 should be no higher than 200)
    C) Always question: Was mask on patient, cannula in nose, etc.?

5. Check PaO_2/SaO_2 – SpO_2 relationship (See page 69)
    Relationship should correlate. Discrepancies indicate a problem with
    the ABG sample (sampling time delay, venous blood, air in sample,
    leukocyte larcency, etc.) or a problem with the pulse oximeter read-
    ing.

6. Check PaO_2 – $PaCO_2$ Relationship
    On room air and at normal atmospheric pressure: The combined PaO_2
    and $PaCO_2$ should never read > 150 mmHg.

**For assessment of quality of test and validity of results,
see AARC Evidence-Based Guideline on next page.**

Blood Gas Analysis and Hemoximetry[1]
(AARC Reference-Based Guidelines Selected Summary)

Indications

Adequacy of ventilation, acid-base, oxygenation status, including oxygen-carry capacity and intrapulmonary shunt

Quantify response to therapeutic intervention or diagnostics

Monitor severity and progression of disease processes

Assess inadequacy of circulatory response

When ABG can't be obtained:
Central Venous or Capillary samples are preferable

Contraindications

Improperly functioning or insufficiently tested/maintained equipment

Improper specimen (anti-coagulation, air bubbles).

Time Sample Sits:
> 30 mins at room temp
> 5 mins at room temp for shunt study
↑ Leukocytes or Platelets - sample must be cooled immediately (↓ PaO_2 rapidly)

Lack of or insufficient acquisition and documentation

Unlabeled specimen

Hazards

Exposure to blood

Inappropriate medical treatments if results are inaccurate

Possible Errors

Clotting

Contamination by air, excess anticoagulant, saline

Inadvertent venous sample

Delay in sample analysis

Inappropriate collection and handling (mixing sample, sample size, etc.)

Dyshemoglobins present

Excess fetal hemoglobin

Transport by tube (under- or over-estimates PO_2)

Quality Control of Analyzer

Errors with VBG:

Use with COPD for pH, HCO_3, but not PO_2, PCO_2

DO NOT use in COPD-exacerbation or acute trauma

DO NOT use with neo seizure, shock, CHF, Congenital Heart Diseases

---

1) Adapted from the AARC Evidence-Based Guidelines: Blood Gas Analysis and Hemoximetry, *Respiratory Care*, 2013.

Oakes' ABG Pocket Guide

Oxygen Therapy for Adults in the Acute Care Facility[1] (AARC Reference-Based Guidelines)

Indications

Acute MI

Hypoxemia (actual or suspected)

  $PaO_2 < 60$ mm Hg
  $SaO_2 < 90\%$
  (or below desired) in adults, children, infants > 28 days in room air.

Severe trauma

Short-term therapy or postop

Precautions/Complications

Ventilatory depression: patients on an O_2 drive with elevated $PaCO_2$ and $PaO_2 \geq 60$ mm Hg.

$FIO_2 > 0.5$: absorption atelectasis, ↓ciliary function, ↓leukocyte function, fire hazard, bacterial contamination (humidification system), caution in patients with paraquat poisoning or receiving bleomycin, O_2 toxicity.

Contraindications

Monitoring

Patient:

  Clinical assessment (pulm, CV, neuro status)

  PaO_2 and/or SaO_2:
    Upon initiation of therapy or within –
      2 hours (COPD)
      8 hours ($FIO_2 > 0.4$)
      12 hours ($FIO_2 < 0.4$)
      72 hours (acute MI)

Equipment:

  Every day or more freq. when: $FIO_2 > 0.5$, clinically unstable, heated gas mixture, artificial airway, blending systems.

Frequency

Continuous or intermittent (exercise, sleep)

1) Adapted from the AARC Clinical Practice Guidelines: Oxygen Therapy for Adults in the Acute Care Facility, 2002 Revision & Update *Respiratory Care*, Volume 47, #6, 2002.

Other Recommended Guidelines

AARC Expert Panel Reference-Based Guidelines:

- Transcutaneous Blood Gas Monitoring for Neonatal and Pediatric Patients
- Capnography/Capnometry During Mechanical Ventilation
- Oxygen Therapy in the Home or Alternate Site Health Care Facility
- Capillary Blood Gas Sampling for Neonatal and Pediatric Patients

Each of these are available in full text at www.rc.joural.com/cpgs

notes:

notes:

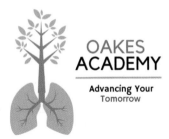

STEPS OF ABG INTERPRETATION

A. Classification   *(See chart next page)*

Primary Problem

Step 1	Check pH - Acidosis or Alkalosis?

Primary Cause

Step 2	Check $PaCO_2$ - Is Respiratory the primary cause?

Step 3	Check HCO_3 - Is Metabolic the primary cause?

Compensation

Step 4	Is the Body Compensating?

Initial Classification

Step 5	Technical / Functional Classifications

B. Calculations

Step 6	Determine Compensation / Other Primary Causes

	$PaCO_2$	pH	HCO_3	Quick Reference Charts:
Respiratory Acidosis				
Acute	↑ 10	↓ 0.08	↑ 1*	See page 31
Chronic	↑ 10	↓ 0.03	↑ 4	
Respiratory Alkalosis				
Acute	↓ 10	↑ 0.08	↓ 2*	See page 44
Chronic	↓ 10	↑ 0.03	↓ 5	

	HCO_3	pH †	$PaCO_2$ ‡	Quick Reference
Metabolic Acidosis	↓ 1	↓ 0.015	↓ 1.2	See page 50
Metabolic Alkalosis	↑ 1	↑ 0.015	↑ 0.7	See page 58

Step 7	Determine Anion Gap and Bicarbonate Gap

a. Anion Gap: $AG = Na - (Cl + HCO_3)$

b. Bicarbonate Gap (if an AG acidosis):

$BG = $ Patient's $HCO_3 + \Delta AG$

BG Norm $= 24 = $ AG Metabolic Acidosis

$< 20 = $ AG Met. Acidosis + Non AG Met. Acidosis

$> 28 = $ AG Met. Acidosis + Met. Alkalosis